PRACTICAL CT TECHNIQUES

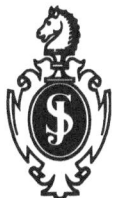

PRACTICAL CT
TECHNIQUES

Wladyslaw Gedroyc and Sheila Rankin

With 38 Figures

Springer-Verlag
London Berlin Heidelberg New York
Paris Tokyo Hong Kong
Barcelona Budapest

Wladyslaw Gedroyc, FRCR
Consultant Radiologist, Department of Diagnostic Radiology,
St. Mary's Hospital, Praed Street, London W2 1NY, UK

Sheila Rankin, FRCR
Consultant Radiologist, Department of Radiology,
Guy's Hospital, St. Thomas Street, London SE1 9RT, UK

ISBN 978-3-540-19726-3 ISBN 978-1-4471-3275-2 (eBook)
DOI 10.1007/978-1-4471-3275-2

British Library Cataloguing in Publication Data
Gedroyc, Wladyslaw
    Practical CT Techniques
I. Title II. Rankin, Sheila
616.07
ISBN 978-3-540-19726-3

Library of Congress Cataloging in Publication Data
Gedroyc, Wladyslaw, 1954–
    Practical CT techniques/Wladyslaw Gedroyc and Sheila Rankin
        p. cm.
ISBN 978-3-540-19726-3
1. Tomography. I. Rankin, Sheila, 1948– . II. Title.
[DNLM: 1. Tomography, X-Ray Computed–methods. WN 160 G296p]
RC78.7.T6G4 1992
616.07'572–dc20
DNLM/DLC   91-47736
for Library of Congress   CIP

Typeset by Fox Design, Surbiton, Surrey

28/3830-543210 Printed on acid-free paper

PREFACE

CT scanners have become an integral part of radiology departments in most hospitals in this country over the last 5 years. They are no longer machines which are confined to larger specialist centres, but have become everyday diagnostic workhorses solving a wide variety of diagnostic problems. As a result most radiologists and radiographers now have to be familiar with all aspects of this technology, its strengths and weaknesses, and the problems of carrying out the scanning sequence most appropriate to the clinical problem being investigated.

This book is an attempt to provide some practical, simple guidelines for scanning most of the areas of the body that CT can be applied to. The various aspects of a successful scan that need to be considered such as patient preparation, slice thickness, i.v. contrast etc., are fully described in a consistent format to allow easy cross reference throughout the book.

We believe that this book will be of most use to radiographers working with CT and to student radiographers being introduced to CT. Junior radiologists working with CT for the first time should also find this book a useful introduction.

A small volume like this cannot be comprehensive and there are inevitably many other methods available for scanning the areas described, which will produce equally satisfactory results. Our intention is that the sequences and protocols described here will provide a sound basis that can be changed and adapted as appropriate to suit your own requirements.

December 1991

Wladyslaw Gedroyc
Sheila Rankin

CONTENTS

INTRODUCTION AND GLOSSARY

This short text is not a recipe book, but rather some suggested protocols for CT scanning. These act as a starting point only and should be altered depending on the clinical problem and the type of CT scanner available. The terminology used with the different machines is very variable. Below is a list of the terminology used in this text, each with a definition.

Patient preparation. Nil by mouth for 2 h is recommended if intravenous contrast is to be given, in case the patient vomits, and nil by mouth for 4 h if oral contrast is to be given, as the patient needs to drink a large volume (800 ml), which is difficult on a full stomach. Obviously scans can be performed on unprepared patients if required.

Slice thickness. Routine slice width is 10 mm. This may vary from 8 mm to 10 mm, depending on the manufacturer. The other slice widths we use in this text are 1.5 mm, 3 mm, and 5 mm.

Slice incrementation is the table movement. Therefore, if the slice thickness is 10 mm and the incrementation is 15 mm, 5 mm of the patient will not be scanned. Contiguous scans have no gap between them.

Interscan delay is the time between the beginning of one scan and the beginning of the next. The shortest times will be when the images are not reconstructed or archived, and it is then the scan time and time for table movement.

Dynamic scanning. This is when scans are taken with the shortest interscan delay, often with the images processed at the end of the sequence. No table movement between scans.

Dynamic incremental scanning. This is the same as above, but with table incrementation.

Scanogram. This is the planning scan of the patient from which slice positions are selected. Also called plan scan, scout view topogram or scanogram, depending on the manufacturer.

High-resolution scan. A thin-section scan with more measurement profiles than a regular scan for increased spatial resolution. Longer scan time. Increased mAs.

Precision scan. A scan with a higher mA for larger patients, or for areas where there are excessive overlying structures such as the shoulders. Unless otherwise stated a regular scan is used.

Reconstruction algorithms. Most scanners have between three and seven algorithms, from smooth to bone. In this text we assume there are seven, 1 being very smooth and 7 bone.

Reformat. Computer reconstruction of transaxial scan data to produce coronal, sagittal, oblique and para-oblique scans.

Window settings. These are a personal preference. However, for ease of comparison between different scans on the same patient, constant values should be used. Remember that lesions often become more obvious with narrow windows; this is very important when viewing the liver. Conversely, wide window widths will obscure lesions – especially important in the head.

WW - Window width. The range of Hounsfield units to be allocated.

WL - Window level. The centre of this range.

HU - Hounsfield units.

ABDOMEN

Patient Preparation

Nil by mouth for 4 h before. Oral contrast is given to opacify the small bowel and stomach, to help differentiate it from pathological masses, which may be of similar attenuation and difficult to separate from bowel.
A suggested mixture is 800 ml water mixed with 16 ml of either meglumine/sodium diatrizoate (gastrografin, urografin) or similar contrast, to make a 2% solution of contrast. To make the urografin palatable, orange or other fruit squash should be added to taste. A dilute proprietary barium solution (EZ-CAT) can be used instead, made up as directed. A cup of the contrast is kept aside and the remainder is given to the patient 30–40 min prior to the scan. The final cup is taken immediately before the scan. This should ensure that the stomach and proximal small bowel are filled.

Patient Position

Supine with the arms above the head. The scans are usually taken on suspended respiration, often on expiration. Suspended inspiration may be used, especially if following a chest CT that has been performed on inspiration. If very short scan times are used, quiet breathing may be more suitable, although not usually in

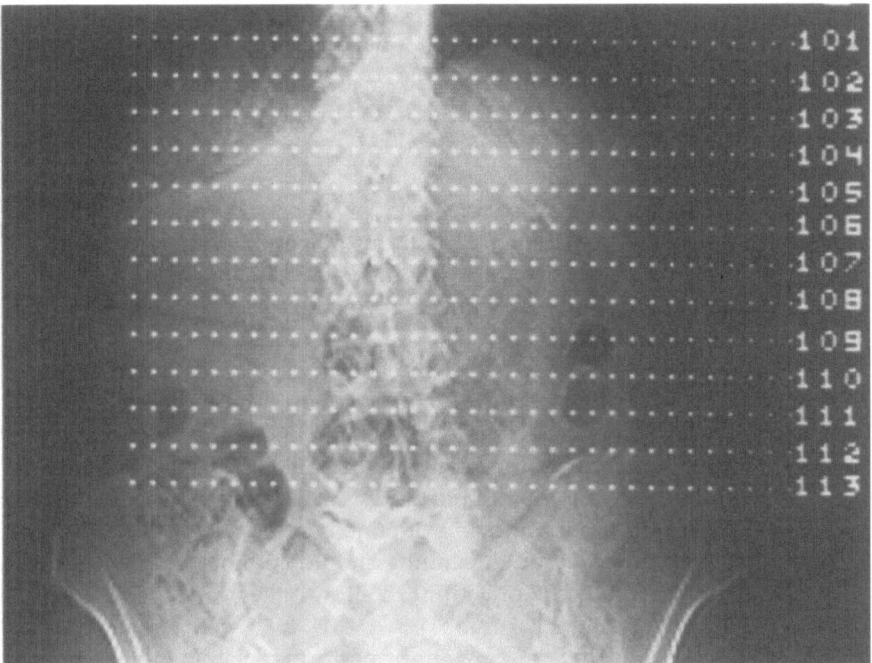

Fig. 1 AP scout. Scan from dome of diaphragm to L5.

the upper abdomen, where respiratory excursion is often maximal. If the duodenal C-loop has been poorly filled, turn the patient into the right lateral decubitus position, giving more oral contrast if the stomach is empty, and this will fill the loop.

Scan Parameters

Frontal abdominal scanogram (Fig. 1). If the scanner has a variable length scanogram or scout view, use the shortest one appropriate for the area to be scanned, particularly in children. Scan from the dome of the diaphragm to the aortic bifurcation (L5).

Slice Thickness: 10 mm

Slice Incrementation: 15 mm if a survey is to be performed, and 10 mm through the area of interest. For better definition of abnormalities a 5 mm slice should be used and contiguous scans obtained (i.e. 5 mm incrementation).

Field of View: 32 cm or 40 cm depending on the size of the patient. A 48 cm or 50 cm field may be required if the entire body outline is to be included; this is often required for radiotherapy planning.

I.V. Contrast: If the abdominal vessels are to be demonstrated, 50–100 cc of intravenous contrast should be given. To perform dynamic incremental scanning, a rapid injection of a loading bolus of 25 ml is given, followed by the remainder of the contrast injected while the scans are being obtained (up to 120 s, depending on the machine). Scanning should commence 20 s after the start of the injection, to allow opacification of the abdominal aorta.

If the scanner cannot perform dynamic incremental scanning, or only a few scans can be obtained before tube cooling delays occur, then repeated smaller doses of contrast at multiple levels may be required.

Window Settings: The abdomen can be viewed with the level (WL) approximately 10% of the window width (WW). Suggested values are WW 400 HU and WL 40 HU, or WW 300 HU and WL 30 HU. For improved contrast resolution, especially in the liver, a narrow window width of 200 HU with a decreased window level may be advantageous. As the lung bases are included in the scan, lung windows (WW 800–1000 HU, WL –800 HU) can be taken, especially if the scan is for suspected malignancy, as lung metastases frequently occur at the bases.

GASTRIC CANCER

Oral Contrast: The final 200 ml are given immediately before scanning, to ensure that the stomach is fully distended in order to assess wall thickness. Gas tablets and paralysis of the stomach, and positioning as for a double-contrast barium study, may be helpful to assess specific areas of the wall. If only the stomach is to be assessed, 600 ml of water can be used as the contrast, with gastric paralysis (Buscopan (hyoscine butylbromide) 20 mg i.v.).

Slice Thickness: 10 mm. 5 mm through area of interest for better spatial resolution.

Slice Incrementation: 10 mm through the liver and stomach, 15 mm to the bifurcation (L5).

Field of View: 32 cm or 40 cm.

I.V. Contrast: May be given initially as for dynamic incremental scanning (see above), to assess the liver and differentiate nodes from coeliac vessels, or after precontrast scans to elucidate specific problems.

Window Settings: See abdomen. WW 400 HU, WL 40 HU.

LYMPHOMA

Oral Contrast: As abdomen.

Slice Thickness: 10 mm.

Slice Incrementation: 15 mm to bifurcation or pubic symphysis.

Field of View: 32 cm or 40 cm.

I.V. Contrast: Not usually required initially.

Window Settings: As abdomen – WW 400 HU, WL 40 HU.

TESTICULAR TERATOMA

Oral Contrast: See abdomen.

Slice Thickness: 10 mm.

Slice Incrementation: 15 mm. Diaphragm to symphysis.

Field of View: 32 cm or 40 cm.

I.V. Contrast: Not usually required.

Window Settings: See abdomen – WW 400 HU, WL 40 HU.

ADRENALS

Patient Preparation

Nil by mouth for 4 h before. 400 ml of oral contrast is usually sufficient given 20 min prior to the scan, as only the bowel in the upper abdomen needs to be opacified. The empty fundus of the stomach may occasionally be mistaken for a left adrenal mass, so ensure that the stomach is full of contrast.

Patient Position

Supine with the arms above the head. Scans should be performed in expiration.

Scan Parameters

Frontal abdominal scanogram (Fig. 2). Scan from just below the right hemidiaphragm to the level of the left renal hilum (L2). The right adrenal is above the right kidney, whereas the left adrenal lies anterior to the upper pole of the left kidney. When screening for phaeochromocytomas, scans should be continued through the retroperitoneum down to the organ of Zuckerkandel, around the origin of the inferior mesenteric artery, at the level of L3.

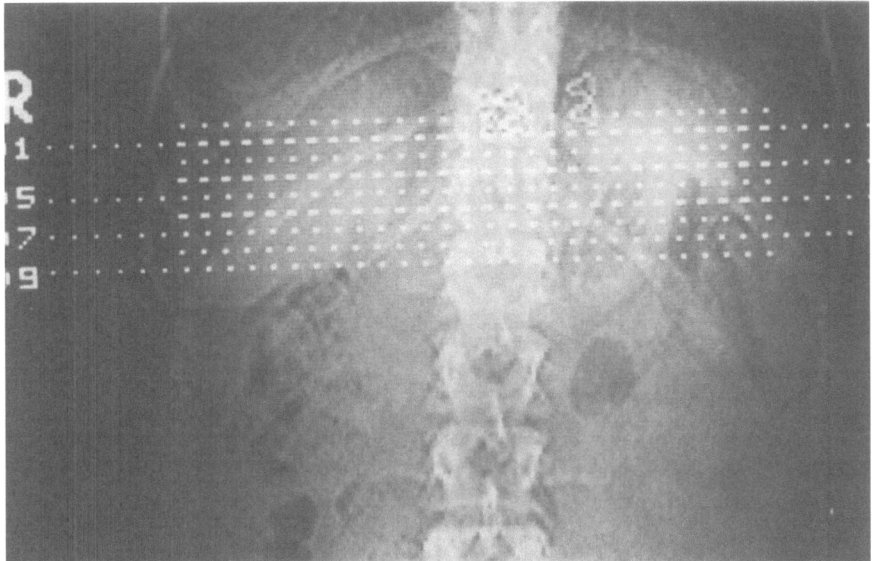

Fig. 2 AP scout. Scan from below diaphragm to L2.

Slice Thickness: 5 mm.

Slice Incrementation: 5 mm.

Field of View: 24 cm.

I.V. Contrast: This is not routinely required, but may be helpful in an attempt to characterise adrenal masses. It may be contraindicated if a phaeochromocytoma is suspected, because of the theoretical risk of a hypertensive reaction, although this is very rare in reality.

Window Settings: WW 400 HU, WL 40 HU.

Measurements of adrenal size include the thickness of the gland, which should not exceed 10 mm, with each limb measuring less than 5 mm. The anteroposterior dimension is less than 40 mm and the superoinferior extent less than 40 mm.

ANKLES

Patient Position

Supine. Feet first, both feet. For *transaxial scans*: feet flexed to 90°, both feet in similar position. Straps may be required to maintain the position or rest the feet against a wedge. For *coronal scans*: both feet flat on table with the knees flexed, and angle the gantry craniad so that the beam passes through the tibiotalar joint at as close to right-angles as possible.

Scan Parameters

Lateral scanogram. For *transaxial examination* scan from the bottom of the calcaneum craniad through the tibiotalar joint or the area of interest. For a *coronal examination* (Fig. 3) scan from the posterior margin of the tibia to the anterior margin of the talus, or through the area of interest.

Slice Thickness: 3 mm.

Slice Incrementation: 3 mm. Contiguous.

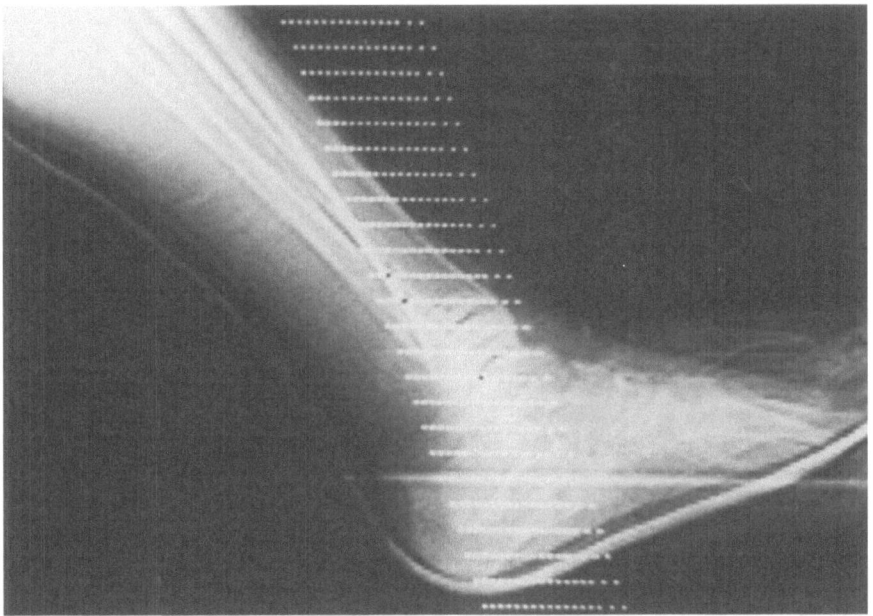

Fig. 3 Lateral scout. Scan from posterior tibia to anterior margin of the talus.

Field of View: If both feet, need 24–32 cm. If one foot, 16–24 cm. High-precision scan. Bone algorithm.

I.V. Contrast: Not usually needed.

Window Settings: Soft tissue WW 400 HU, WL 40 HU; bone WW 3200 HU, WL 200 HU.

Tarsal Coalition: Transaxial.

Loose Bodies: Coronal.

Avascular Necrosis: Coronal.

Subtalar Joints: Coronal.

AORTA

THORACIC AORTIC ANEURYSM

Patient Preparation

Nil by mouth for 2 h before.

Patient Position

Supine with the arms above the head. Scan on suspended inspiration. With very short scan times and interscan delays it may be better to scan on quiet shallow respiration.

Scan Parameters

Frontal chest scanogram. Scan from just above the aortic arch down to below the diaphragm, and continuing to below the aortic bifurcation (L5) if the aorta remains aneurysmal.

Slice Thickness: 10 mm.

Slice Incrementation: 15 mm.

Field of View: 32 cm for the whole body or 24 cm if limited to the aorta.

I.V. Contrast: 50–100 ml of warm contrast. Dynamic incremental scans are performed with the minimum interscan delay, so that the contrast levels in the aorta remain as high as possible throughout the scans. 25–50 ml of contrast are given as a bolus, and the remainder given while the scans are obtained. This will take up to 90–120 s, depending on the number of scans and the interscan delay. A hand injection or a pressure injector, which is preferable, can be used. Non-ionic contrast is preferred as there is usually less patient movement due to nausea. Start scanning 5 s after commencing the injection.

Window Settings: WW 400 HU, WL 40 HU.

ABDOMINAL AORTIC ANEURYSM

Patient Preparation

Nil by mouth for 2 h before. 400 ml of oral contrast 30 min before. The extra cup of contrast is not required as the stomach does not need to be full. The oral contrast is required in case there is either an inflammatory aneurysm or other retroperitoneal disease, rather than a simple aneurysm. In an emergency, for example a bleeding aneurysm, the oral contrast can be omitted.

Patient Position

Supine with the arms above the head. Suspended respiration if possible. In very sick patients with multiple lines the arms may have to be down, but avoid

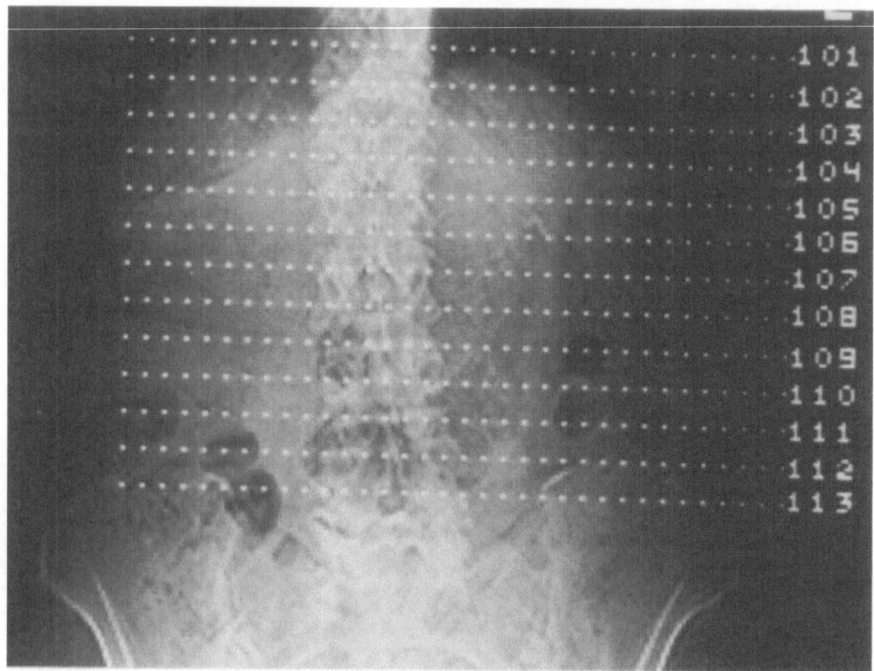

Fig. 4 AP scout. Scan from dome of diaphragm to L5.

this if possible because of the artefact generated. If necessary have only one arm above the head.

Scan Parameters

Frontal abdominal scanogram. Scan from the top of the kidneys (L1) or the diaphragm to the aortic bifurcation (L5), and continue down to the pubic symphysis if the iliac arteries are to be visualised (Fig. 4).

Slice Thickness: 10 mm. A 5 mm scan with consequent improved spatial resolution may be preferred at the level of the renal arteries, to ascertain the relationship of the renal arteries to the aortic aneurysm. These can always be done at the end of the procedure when the origin of the arteries has been localised.

Slice Incrementation: 15 mm, except at the level of the renal hilus (L2) when the slices should be contiguous, to define the relationship of the renal arteries to the aneurysm.

I.V. Contrast: 50–100 ml of warm contrast, given as above, but start scanning 20 s after the injection commences. If the scanner cannot perform enough scans because of tube cooling limitations then multiple boluses of 25–40 ml may be required.

Window Settings: WW 400 HU, WL 40 HU. Sometimes a narrower WW of 300 HU may be helpful.

DISSECTING AORTIC ANEURYSM

Patient Preparation

None. Nil by mouth for 2 h before if time permits.

Patient Position

As above. It is important to move all metallic objects out of the way as they cause artefacts across the aorta that may be mistaken for an intimal flap.

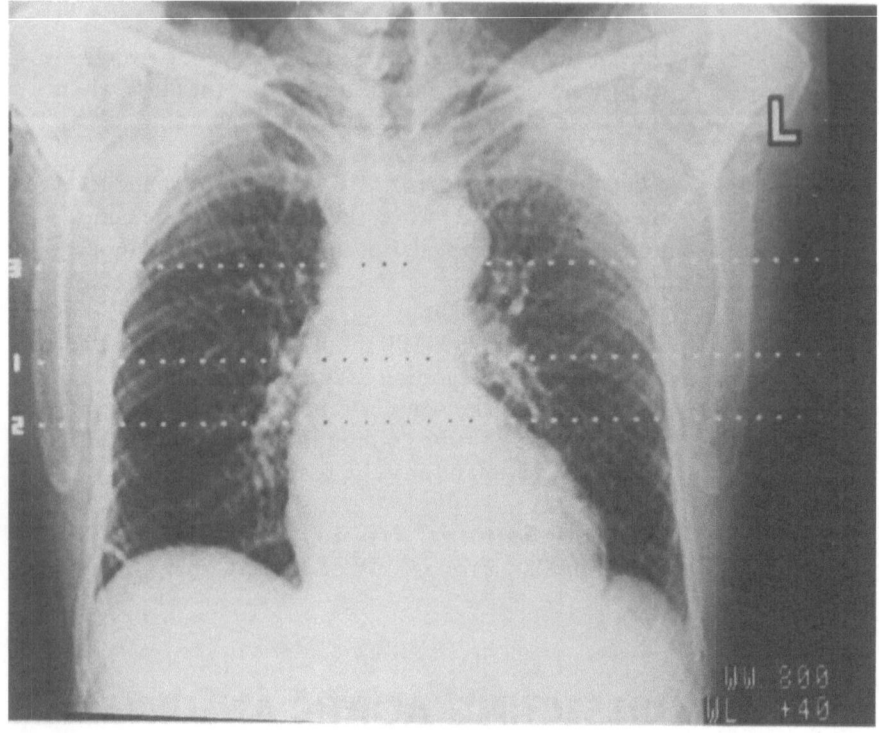

Fig. 5 AP scout. Scan at aortic root, mid-ascending aorta and across the aortic arch.

Scan Parameters

Frontal chest scanogram (Fig. 5). Three levels are chosen; at each level dynamic scanning without table incrementation is performed. A level is chosen and 40 ml of contrast is injected as rapidly as possible, and five or six scans are obtained immediately after the injection. These are viewed and the next level is then chosen and the procedure repeated.

1st Level: Just above the aortic valve.

2nd Level: In mid-ascending aorta.

3rd Level: Across the arch of the aorta. If the first scan shows a dissection involving both the ascending and the descending aorta, then the second scan in the mid-ascending aorta can be omitted. The scan across the arch should still be performed, in an attempt to separate the rare type III dissection that dissects both distally and proximally from its entry point distal to the left subclavian, to involve both the ascending and the descending aorta, from a type I dissection which involves the ascending and the descending aorta, entering just above the aortic valve (type I). If a type III dissection is diagnosed, its distal extent should be assessed and dynamic incremental scanning should be performed through the chest and abdomen as for thoracic aneurysms (see above).

Slice Thickness: 10 mm.

Slice Incrementation: None. If scanning the remainder of the chest and abdomen, 15 mm.

Field of View: 32 cm.

I.V. Contrast: 40 ml warmed non-ionic contrast given as a bolus, as hard and as fast as possible if a hand injection. If a pressure injector is used, give at 8–10 ml/s. Scanning should commence 5 s after the contrast starts, so that the contrast can be watched as it passes through the true and the false lumens.

Window Settings: WW 400 HU, WL 40 HU. Narrower window widths of 200–300 HU may be helpful when assessing the intimal flap, particularly if there is artefact from pacemakers or cardiac motion.

Bladder

Patient Preparation

Nil by mouth for 4 h before. 800 ml of oral contrast (see abdomen) is given 1 h before, to allow all the small bowel to be filled. For better and guaranteed filling of the small bowel, give a mixture of 800 ml water, 50 ml 70% sorbitol and 30 ml urografin with orange squash to taste. Give 200 ml every 15 min, with the last cup given 15 min before scanning. The sorbitol acts as an osmotic load, drawing water into the bowel and decreasing transit time. This mixture produces excellent filling of the small bowel, and usually the colon, within an hour, but may cause severe transient diarrhoea about 90 min after starting the contrast – the patient should be warned. Rectal contrast may be required if sorbitol is not used. Full bladder.

Patient Position

Supine with the arms above the head. Scan on suspended expiration.

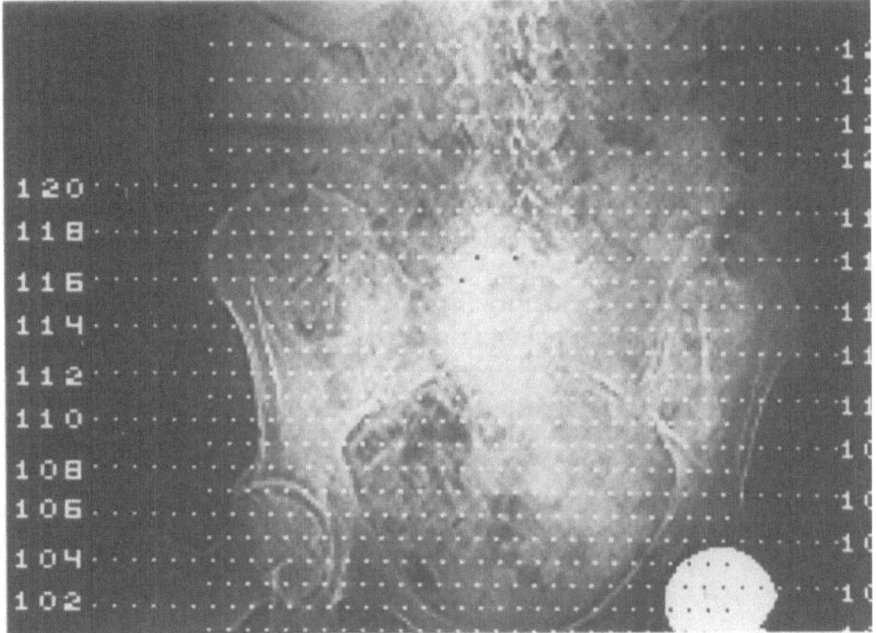

Fig. 6 AP scout. Scan from pubic symphysis to mid-kidneys.

Scan Parameters

Frontal abdominal scanogram (Fig. 6) to include the abdomen and pelvis. Scan from the symphysis to at least the mid-kidneys, or the diaphragm if the liver is to be included.

Slice Thickness: 10 mm. For better definition of the bladder wall, 5 mm contiguous scans through the bladder on a 24 cm field of view may be helpful.

Slice Incrementation: 10 mm through the bladder. 15 mm for the remainder of the abdomen.

Field of View: 32 cm or 40 cm. A smaller 24 cm field if 5 mm thick scans obtained.

I.V. Contrast: Not required for the bladder as the urine acts as a very good contrast agent, and dense contrast may obscure small tumours. Contrast may be helpful in delineating the iliac vessels and separating them from nodes. 50–100 ml of contrast is given, 25–50 ml as a bolus and the remainder while dynamic incremental scans are being performed through the pelvis. Scanning should start least 25 s after the injection begins, to allow time for the contrast to reach the iliac vessels. Delayed scans can be obtained if the contrast-filled ureters need to be visualised. Obstructed urine-filled ureters are easily visualised on CT without the use of intravenous contrast.

Window Settings: WW 400 HU, WL 40 HU.

BRACHIAL PLEXUS

Patient Preparation

None.

Patient Position

Supine with the arms by the sides.

Scan Parameters

Frontal scanogram of lower neck and upper chest
(Fig. 7). Scan from C5 to T2 initially. A high mA
(precision) scan will be required when scanning through
the shoulders, otherwise use a normal-dose scan. A
slightly edge-enhanced algorithm (filter 5) may be
helpful.

Slice Thickness: 5 mm.

Slice Incrementation: 5 mm.

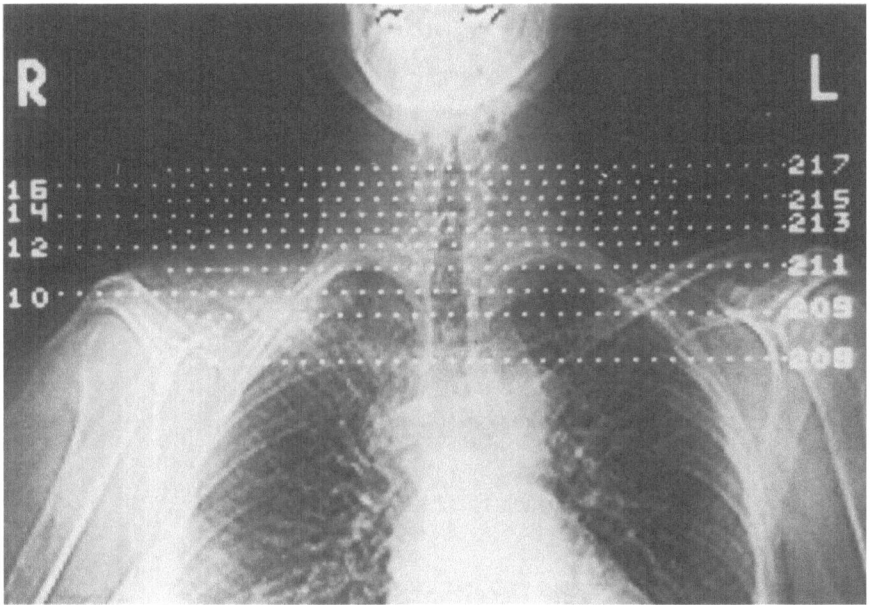

Fig. 7 AP scout. Scan from C5 to T2/3.

Field of View: 16 cm or 24 cm. If the axilla is to be included for patients with breast cancer, use the larger field of view.

I.V. Contrast: Not always required. If contrast is to be given to outline the vessels, perform dynamic incremental scanning using 50 ml of contrast injected into the opposite arm from the side of interest; this will decrease the artefact from the contrast. Start scanning 10 s after commencing the injection.

Window Settings: WW 400 HU, WL 40 HU.

Brain

Patient Preparation

Nil by mouth for 2 h before.

Patient Position

Supine with the head in the headrest provided by the manufacturer, arms by the sides. The chin should be as far down as is comfortably possible, so that the patient will stay in that position. This ensures that a minimum number of scans will pass through the lens.

Scan Parameters

Lateral head scanogram (Fig. 8). Use the shorter length scanogram if available. Scans are taken parallel to the floor of the anterior fossa – the lowest section through the external auditory meatus, and continuing to the top of the head. This normally ensures that the scans avoid the lens. The gantry is angled towards the fleet (negative angulation). To decrease the artefact from beam hardening from the petrous bones across the posterior fossa, a higher mA (precision) scan may be helpful.

Slice Thickness: 5 mm in the posterior fossa, 10 mm for the remainder of the head. In neonates, i.e. less than

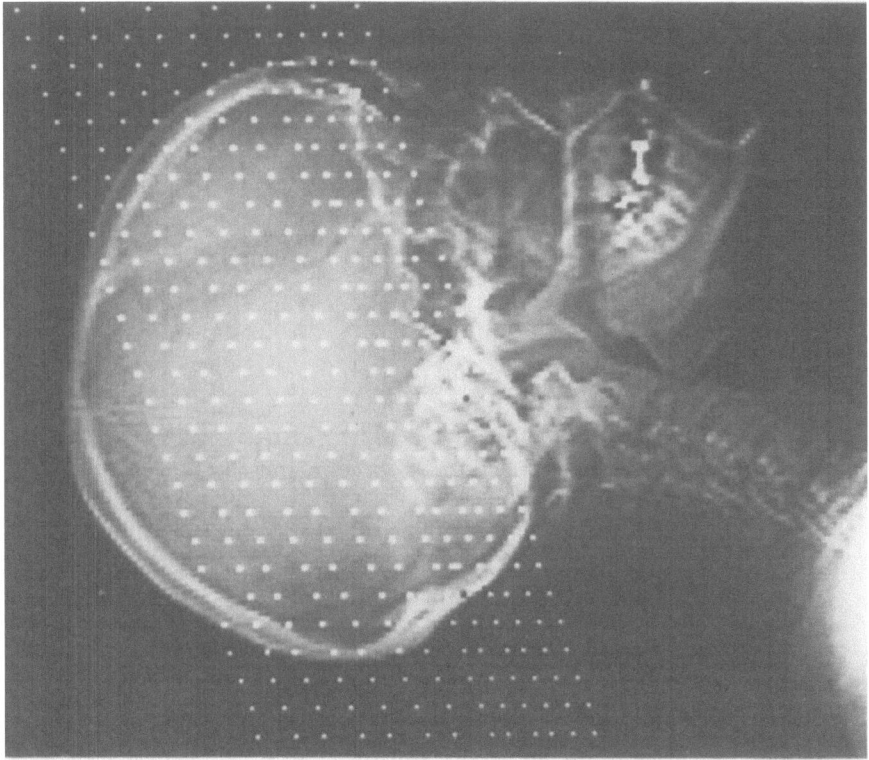

Fig. 8 Lateral scout. Scan from external auditory meatus to vertex.

6 months old, a baby headset (which is low-dose with minimal or no calcium correction) should be used.

Slice Incrementation: Contiguous. 5 mm in the posterior fossa and 10 mm in the remainder.

Field of View: 24 cm.

I.V. Contrast: 50 ml of non-ionic contrast. Not all scans require contrast. Some suggestions for contrast are given below.

Window Settings: Lowest slices through the posterior fossa WW 150 HU, WL 36 HU, decreasing to

WW 100 HU and WL 36 HU through the upper posterior fossa. Above the tentorium WW 75 HU and WL 36 HU. It is important to keep the window settings constant if scans are to be compared.

CLINICAL CONDITIONS

Abscess: Pre- and post-contrast scans.

Aneurysms and Arteriovenous Malformations: Pre- and post-contrast dynamic incremental scans.

Blocked Shunts: Unenhanced scans initially.

Dementia: Unenhanced initially.

Encephalitis: Pre- and post-contrast scans.

Epilepsy: Unenhanced scans initially. If focus is on EEG, enhance.

Temporal Lobe Epilepsy (EEG positive): Precontrast head and a post-contrast scan through the temporal lobes with the patient's chin raised, and scan through the temporal lobes with a reverse angulation of +20°, avoiding the petrous bones and orbits if possible (Fig. 9).

Infarcts: Unenhanced scans only, unless the diagnosis is in doubt. Try to avoid ionic contrast in the first 10 days after the infarct. Try not to scan in the first 4 h after the event, as the infarct, although present, may not be demonstrated and the patient may then require another scan. In order to identify acute haemorrhage, scan within the first 7–10 days, as after this the blood may not be visualised.

Lymphoma: Pre- and post-contrast scans.

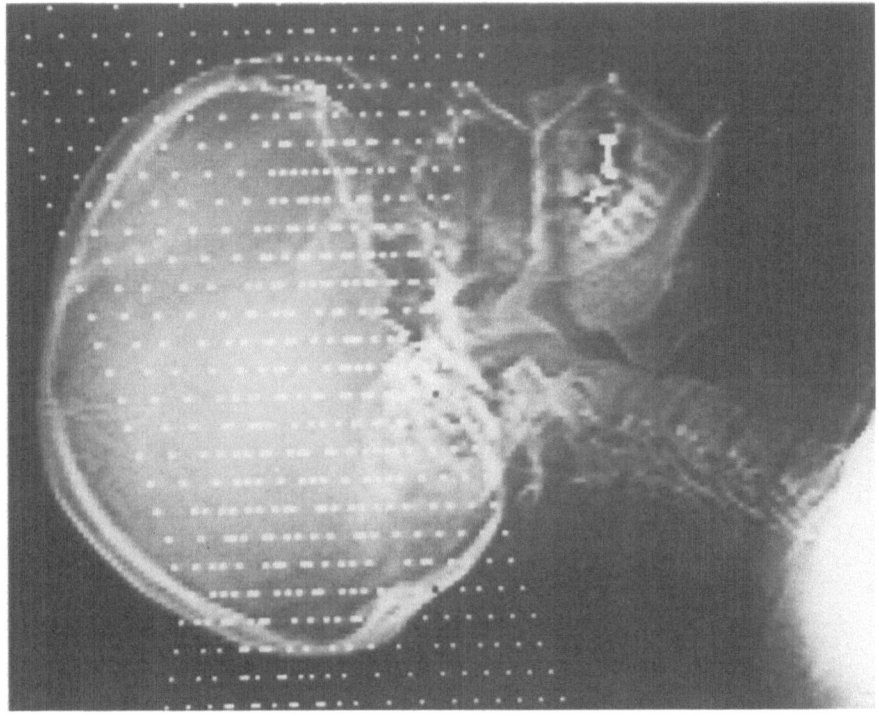

Fig. 9 Lateral scout. Reverse angulation through the temporal lobes.

Meningitis: Pre- and post-contrast scans.

Metastases: Post-contrast only initially. Repeat without contrast if necessary.

Multiple Sclerosis: Unenhanced scan. Contrast *may* demonstrate areas of active demyelination, particularly if delayed scans are obtained.

Trauma: Unenhanced only.

Tumours: Pre- and post-contrast.

Subdural Haematomas: Unenhanced initially. If there is any doubt give contrast, as this will enhance the membrane between the collection and the brain.

CHEST

Patient Preparation

Nil by mouth for 2 h before.

Patient Position

Supine with the arms above the head. Scans are taken on inspiration. Try to ensure that the patient takes the same depth of breath each time, so that all the lung is included in the scan.

Scan Parameters

Frontal chest scanogram. (Fig. 10). Scan from the lung apices to the bottom of the lungs.

Slice Thickness: 10 mm.

Slice Incrementation: 15 mm if survey, otherwise 10 mm.

Field of View: 32 cm or 40 cm.

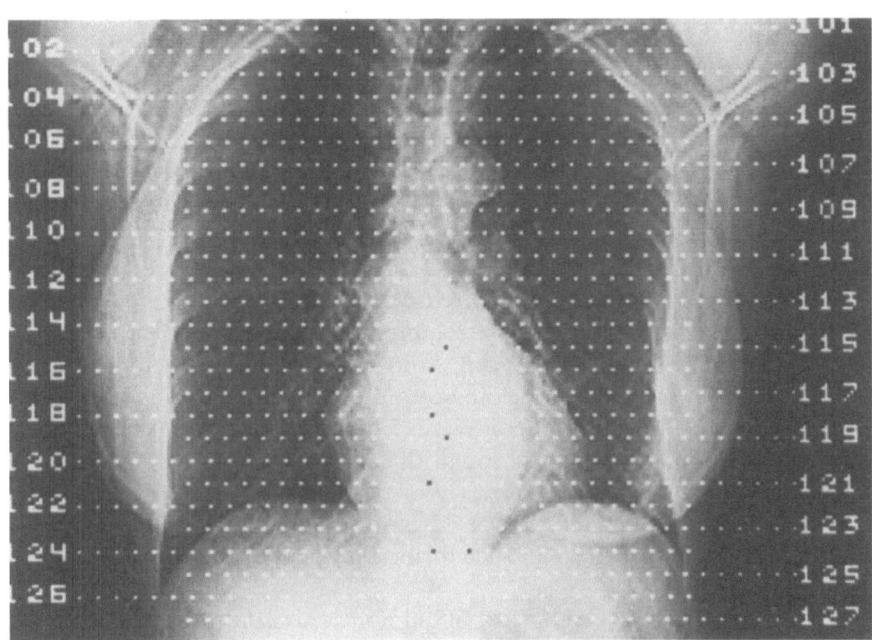

Fig. 10 AP scout. Scan from apex to bottom of the lungs.

I.V. Contrast: May be required to identify vessels. 100 ml of contrast, 25 ml given as a bolus and the remainder given over 90–120 s, or the time taken for the number of scans required, while dynamic incremental scanning is performed. If contrast is given to identify a specific abnormality, 50 ml may be adequate. Start to scan at least 5 s after beginning to inject, as this is the arm–heart transit time with a normal cardiac output.

Window Settings: For mediastinum: WW 400 HU, WL 40 HU. For lung parenchyma: WW 600–800 HU, WL –800 to –1000 HU. To visualise the mediastinum and lung parenchyma together, either use a double window or WW 1000 HU and WL –800 HU.

LUNG CANCER

Scan from apices to bottom of adrenals (L2).

Slice Thickness: 10 mm. Use 5 mm for better detail through the carina and bronchi.

Slice Incrementation: 10 mm contiguous, with contrast given as required. If the number of scans is to be limited, 15 mm from apex of lungs, 10 mm from the aortic arch to the bottom of the carina during the injection of contrast, 15 mm to the bottom of the lungs and 10 mm through the adrenals (L1).

Field of View: 32 cm or 40 cm. 24 cm field of view with a 5 mm slice for better detail of the major bronchi.

I.V. Contrast: 50 ml non-ionic contrast as a bolus, from the aortic arch to the pulmonary veins during dynamic incremental scanning.

Window Settings: As above.

METASTASES

Scan from the lung apices to the bases.

Slice Thickness: 10 mm.

Slice Incrementation: 10 mm.

Field of View: 32 cm or 40 cm.

I.V. Contrast: Not required.

Window Settings: As above.

LYMPHOMA

Scan from the lung apices to the lung bases.

Slice Thickness: 10 mm.

Slice Incrementation 15 mm.

Field of View: 32 cm or 40 cm.

I.V. Contrast: If necessary.

TERATOMA OR SEMINOMA

Scan from lung apices to the lung bases.

Slice Thickness: 10 mm.

Slice Incrementation: 10 mm.

Field of View: 32 cm or 40 cm.

I.V. Contrast: If necessary.

Window Settings: As above.

MEDIASTINAL MASSES

Scan from apices to base.

Slice Thickness: 10 mm.

Slice Incrementation: 10 mm through the lesion; 15 mm remainder of chest.

Field of View: 32 cm or 40 cm.

I.V. Contrast: 50–100 ml non-ionic contrast through chest during dynamic incremental scanning, or use 50 ml if selected scans only are to be enhanced.

Window Settings: As above.

BRONCHIECTASIS, INTERSTITIAL LUNG DISEASE

There are several ways of performing these scans. A routine chest scan can be performed initially as above, and then selected thin sections can be taken through areas of abnormality; or thin sections with wide incrementation can be taken initially. It may be helpful to take scans prone as well as supine if there is any doubt about the gravitational effect on vessels. For the thin sections:

Slice Thickness: 1–2 mm. High precision.

Slice Incrementation: 10–15 mm.

Field of View: 32 cm, or each lung visualised separately on 16–24 cm.

Reconstruction algorithm: Bone (7).

I.V. Contrast: Not required.

Window Settings: Lung parenchyma: WW 1000 HU, WL –750 to –1000 HU. Mediastinum: WW 600 HU, WL 60 HU.

CONTRAST

I.V. Contrast

Either ionic or non-ionic contrast can be used and is given at the discretion of the radiologist. I.V. contrast can be given as a bolus to elucidate particular problems, rather than as a routine infusion. Thus non-ionic contrast may be used in preference to ionic, as it is injected rapidly, and it is important that there is no patient movement between the unenhanced and the enhanced scans as repeat scans are expensive in radiation, contrast and time. The usual volume for adults is 50–100 ml of contrast containing 370 mg/ml iodine. An alternative regimen is to use larger volumes of more dilute contrast – this is recommended if continuous infusions rather than boluses of contrast are injected, and in this case ionic contrast may be used.

Oral Contrast

The oral contrast used may be either a dilute gastrografin solution or a mixture of urografin and orange juice, which patients may find more palatable. The urografin must be flavoured as it is very bitter if mixed only with water. A proprietary barium mixture for CT, made up as directed, may used as above (EZ-CAT).

Oral contrast is always given for abdominal and pelvic scans unless there is a very pressing clinical contraindication. Method of administration: 800 ml water, 16 ml urografin 370, and orange squash to taste. Take off 1 cup before giving the remainder to the patient 30 min before for an abdominal scan, and 60 min before for a pelvic scan. Give the extra cup immediately before scanning.

Pelvic Preparation

To fill the large bowel, 800 ml of dilute, or 20 ml of undiluted contrast can be given the night before to fill the colon, and a further 800 ml the day of the scan as above, to fill the small bowel and stomach. An alternative method for filling all the small bowel and most of the colon is to use a mixture containing sorbitol: 800 ml of water. 50 ml 70% sorbitol, 30 ml contrast, and orange juice to taste. 200 ml are given every 15 min prior to the scan, with the last dose of contrast 15 min before commencing the scan.

Rectal Contrast

6 ml of urografin 370 in 200 ml of water are given as an enema immediately prior to the scan, and the rectum can be inflated with 50 ml of air.

Vaginal Tampon

This introduces air into the vagina, thus marking its position, which may be helpful.

FACE

Patient Preparation

None.

Patient Position

Supine, arms by the sides. Head in headrest, with chin elevated.

Scan Parameters

Lateral head scanogram (Fig. 11). Straight gantry. Scan through area of interest, or from top of frontal sinuses down to bottom of the mandible. Use of a neonatal headset may give better dosimetry. A slightly edge-enhanced filter (5) is recommended.

Slice Thickness: 5 mm.

Slice Incrementation: 5 mm. Contiguous.

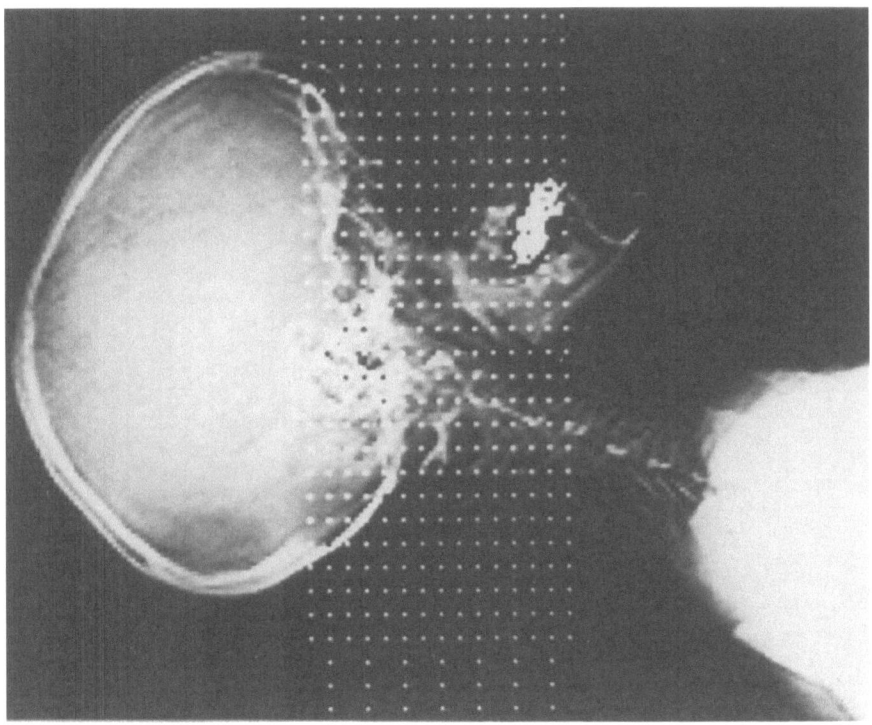

Fig. 11 Lateral scout. Scan from frontal sinus to bottom of mandible.

Field of View: 16 cm and increase to 18 cm if necessary, to include all the soft tissues.

I.V. Contrast: Not normally required.

Window Setting: For soft tissue: WW 400 HU, WL 40 HU. For bone: WW 1600 HU, WL 200 HU.

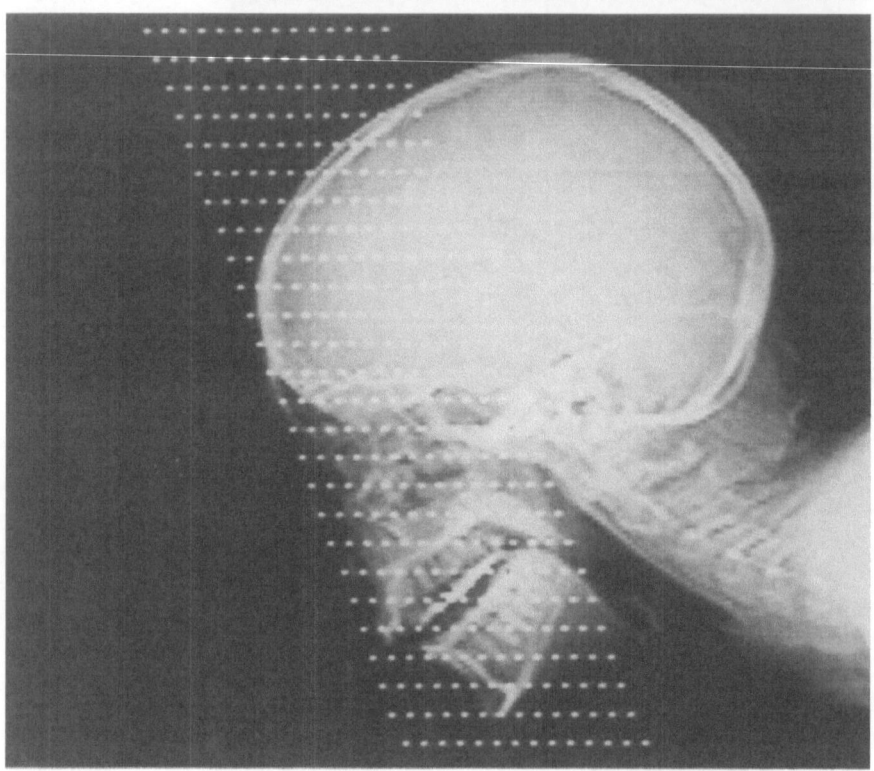

Fig. 12 Coronal scout. Scan perpendicular to the anterior cranial fossa through the face.

Coronal Scans are performed if possible (Fig. 12).

Scan Parameters: Patient prone or supine, depending on the type of coronal headrest supplied by the manufacturer. Lateral scanogram. Angle the gantry so that it is perpendicular to the floor of the anterior cranial fossa. Same scanning parameters as above.

Facial Trauma: Transaxial and coronal if possible.

Facial Tumours: Transaxial and coronal. I.V. contrast is often given, as for the neck, especially if the lymph nodes are to be staged. For nasopharyngeal tumours the base of the skull should be included.

Sinus Disease: If for tumour, transaxial and coronal. If for benign disease, try to do coronal scans only, to decrease the dose to the lens. A 3 mm scan may be required at the level of the ostia for improved spatial resolution. A wider window of 3200 HU may be preferred, so that the mucosa and bone may be visualised together.

Dental Implants: 1–2 mm high-resolution contiguous scans through the maxilla or mandible. Straight gantry. The images are then reformatted perpendicular to the anterior bony surface, and measurements of the depth and thickness of bone are taken.

FEET

Patient Preparation

None.

Patient Position

Supine. Feet first, both feet together in the same position. For coronal scans, feet flat on the table. Transaxial scans, feet dorsiflexed at right angles; it may be helpful to immobilise the feet or rest them against a pad.

Scan Parameters

Lateral scanogram. For transaxial scans, scan parallel to the sole of the foot. For coronal scans, scan perpendicular to the dorsum of the foot and scan the area of interest. Bone algorithm.

Slice Thickness: 3 mm (high resolution) or 5 mm, depending on problem.

Slice Incrementation: Contiguous.

Field of View: 24 cm or 32 cm.

I.V. Contrast: Often not required.

Window Settings: Soft tissue: WW 400 HU, WL 40 HU. Bone: WW 3200 HU, WL 200 HU.

GALLBLADDER

Patient Preparation

No oral contrast. Fast for 12 h before.

Patient Position

Supine with the arms above the head. Scan on suspended expiration.

Scan Parameters

Frontal abdominal scanogram (Fig. 13). Scan from L1 down. The position of the gallbladder is variable and may be intrahepatic, and thus more craniad than this.

Slice Thickness: 5 mm.

Slice Incrementation: 5 mm.

Field of View: 24 cm.

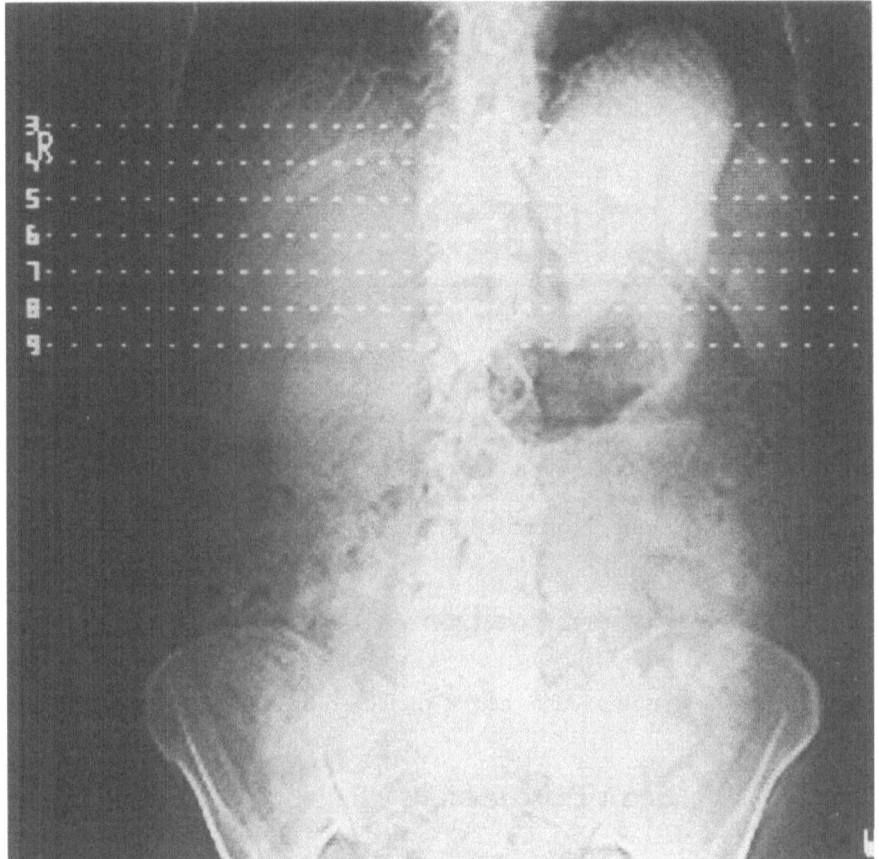

Fig. 13 AP scout. Scan from L1 down.

I.V. Contrast: Not required.

Window Settings: WW 400 HU, WL 40 HU.
A representative Hounsfield value for the bile and for the stones is normally obtained.

Hips

Patient Preparation

None. No oral contrast.

Patient Position

Supine. Arms across the chest. Scan on quiet breathing.

Scan Parameters

Frontal scanogram. Scan from the top of the acetabulum to the bottom of the femoral head. Scans are usually performed after trauma to assess fractures or intra-articular loose bodies. Reformatted images or 3-D reconstruction, if available, may be helpful. If reformatted images are to be obtained, remember not to move the image once scanning has started (Fig. 14).

Slice Thickness: 3 mm. High resolution. Bone algorithm.

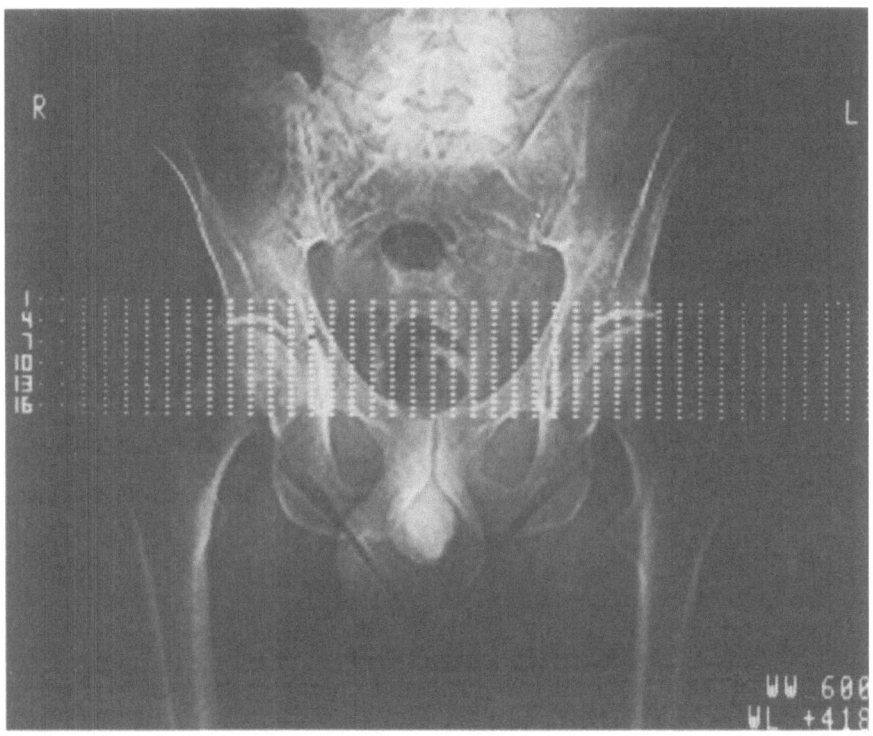

Fig. 14 AP scout. Scan from top of acetabulum to bottom of femoral head.

Slice Incrementation: 3 mm, contiguous.

Field of View: 16 cm if single hip, 32 cm if both hips.

I.V. Contrast: Not required.

Window Settings: Bone: WW 3200 HU, WL 200 HU. Soft tissue: WW 400 HU, WL 40 HU.

INTERNAL AUDITORY MEATUS

Patient Preparation

Nil by mouth for 2 h before.

Patient Position

For transaxial scans, supine with head in headrest supplied. Chin down as for brain scan. For coronal scans, supine or prone, depending on the headrest supplied.

Scan Parameters

Lateral scanogram (Fig. 15). Always transaxial and coronal scans.

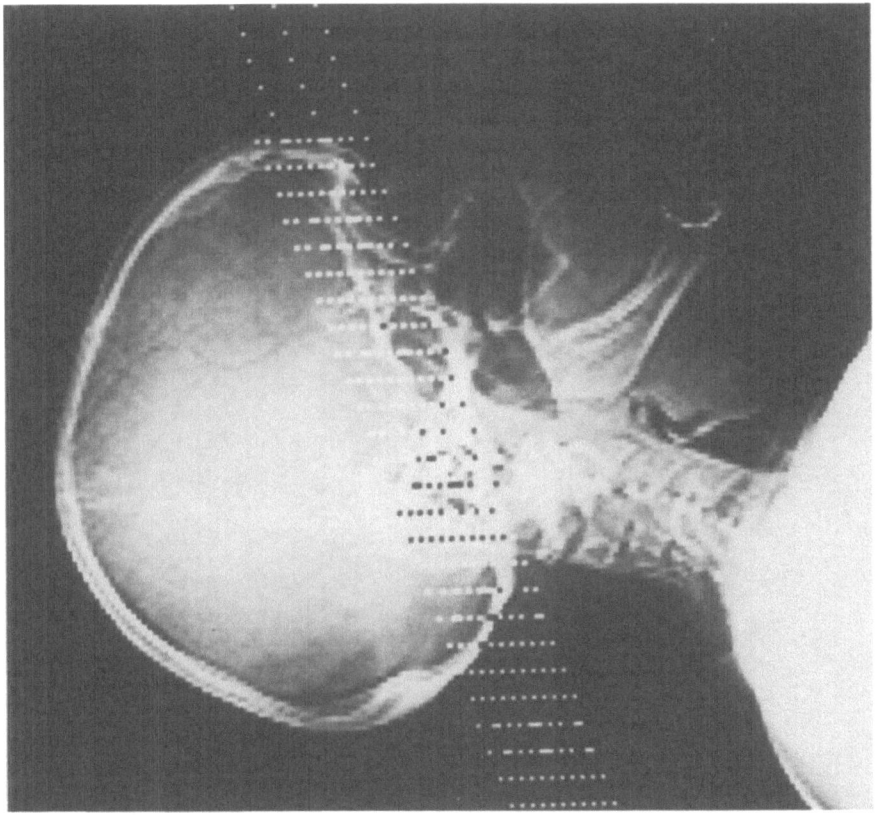

Fig. 15 Lateral scan. Scan from bottom of EAM to the top of the petrous bone.

Transaxial: Scan from below external auditory meatus to top of petrous bone.

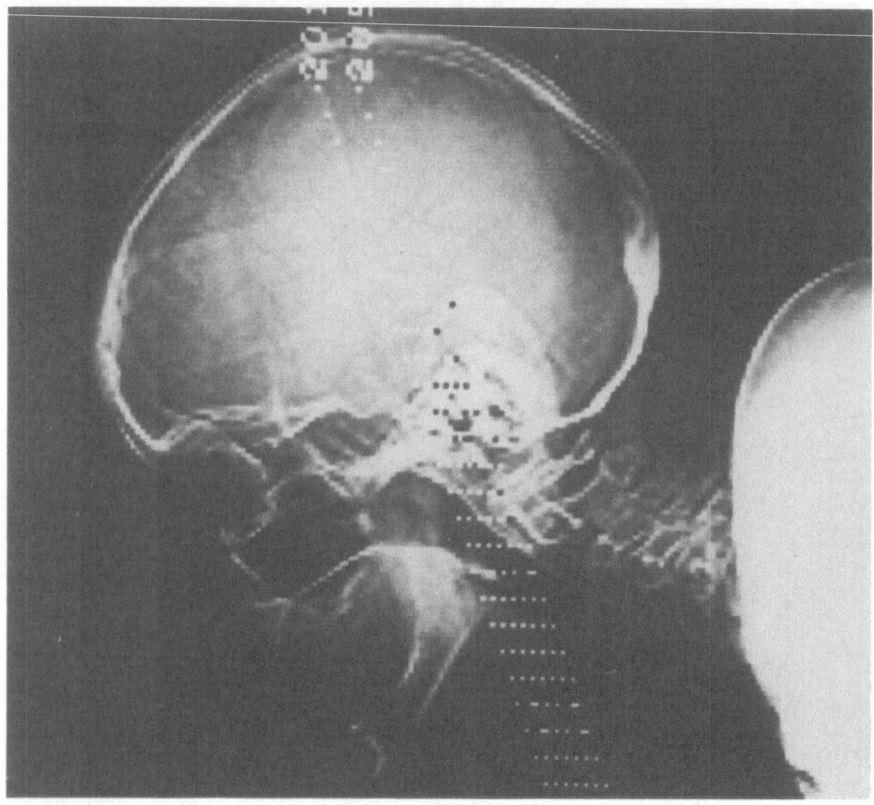

Fig. 16 Lateral scout. Scan from external auditory meatus to the back of the mastoids.

Coronal (Fig. 16): Scan at right-angles to the petrous bones, which usually means angling the gantry + 20°. Scan from the external auditory meatus posteriorly to the back of the mastoids.

Slice Thickness: 3 mm. High resolution.

Slice Incrementation: 3 mm.

Field of View: 24 cm. Can zoom to a single side.

I.V. Contrast: 50 ml of non-ionic contrast. All scans are taken post-contrast only – this decreases the number of scans taken and thus the radiation. If necessary, unenhanced scans can be repeated at a later date. Scans should be reconstructed on both brain and bone algorithms.

Window Settings: Brain: WW 100 HU, WL 36 HU. Bone: WW 3200 HU, WL 200 HU.

KIDNEYS

Patient Preparation

Nil by mouth for 4 h before. Oral contrast as for abdomen.

Patient Position

Patient supine with arms above head. Scan on suspended respiration.

Scan Parameters

Frontal scanogram (Fig. 17). If the kidneys only are to be imaged, scan from T12 to L3. If the whole abdomen is to be included scan from the dome of the diaphragm to the aortic bifurcation (L5).

Slice Thickness: 10 mm. For improved spatial resolution a 5 mm slice may be helpful. Unenhanced scans are usually performed initially.

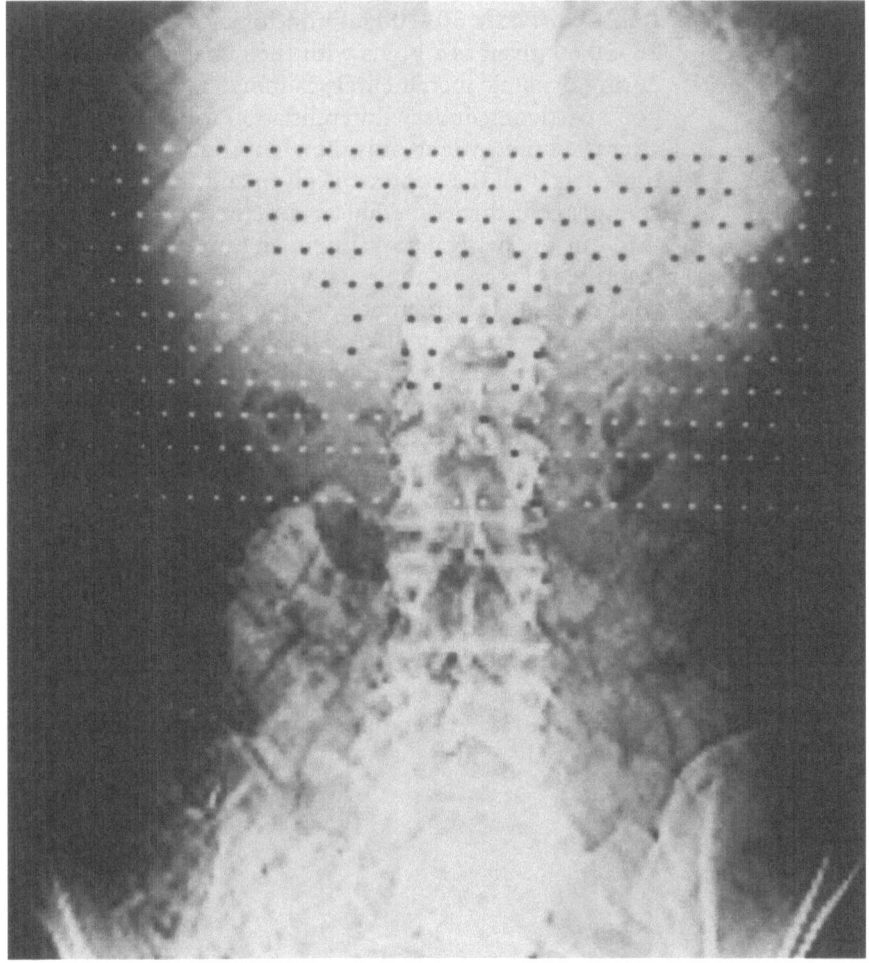

Fig. 17 AP scout. Scan from T12 to L3.

Slice Incrementation: 10 mm, contiguous.

Field of View: 32 cm or 40 cm, depending on size of patient.

I.V. Contrast: 50–100 ml non-ionic contrast, 25–50 ml given as a bolus with the remainder given during dynamic incremental scanning. This gives very good corticomedullary differentiation for the first 30 s after the bolus, which aids the identification of small tumours. If all the contrast is given and then scanning is commenced, corticomedullary differentiation will not be seen but the pelvicaliceal system and ureters will be identified. To assess the renal vein, dynamic scans without table incrementation should be obtained at the level of the renal vein (L2). The first scan should be at least 20 s after the beginning of the bolus injection.

Delayed scans with the patient prone may be helpful in assessing the level of ureteric obstruction, although dilated urine-filled ureters are usually quite easily identified on unenhanced scans.

Renal Calculi: Stones that are non-opaque on conventional films may be identified on CT. Unenhanced scans must be obtained initially, as the i.v. contrast may obscure the calculi.

Renal Cysts: Pre- and post-i.v. contrast as above. Kidneys only.

Renal Tumours: Scan the liver and kidneys with 10 mm contiguous scans pre- and post-i.v. contrast. Give contrast as above and start scanning 20 s after beginning the contrast. Do three scans at the level of the renal vein to exclude tumour thrombus, and then scan the remainder of the liver and kidneys, continuing down to the aortic bifurcation with scan incrementations of 15 mm.

Renal Trauma: Oral contrast. Scan pre- and post-i.v. contrast as above.

Knees

Patient Preparation

None.

Patient Position

Patient supine, feet first into scanner. If both knees are to be imaged, have legs in identical positions even if not straight, as this facilitates anatomic comparison. Knees slightly flexed if this is more comfortable and tie a bandage around ankles to immobilise legs. If only one knee is to be imaged it should be in the centre of the field, with the knee flexed to 8–10° with the contra-lateral leg resting against the gantry housing.

Scan Parameters

Anteroposterior or lateral scanogram, depending on the clinical problem. For patellar alignment usually both knees are scanned and an AP scanogram is obtained. For assessment of the cartilage a lateral scanogram is used (Fig. 18) and the gantry angled parallel to the tibial plateau (positive angulation). The meniscus can be visualised without the use of intra-articular contrast; however, the scan can be performed following a

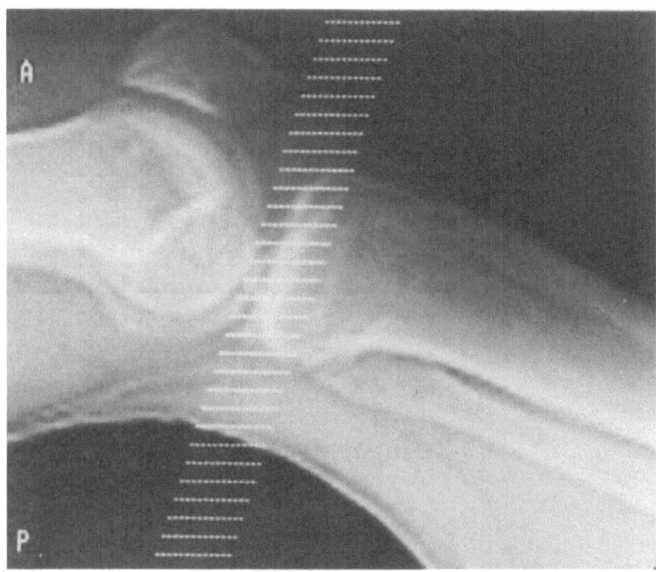

Fig. 18 Lateral scout. Scan parallel to the tibial plateau.

conventional knee arthrogram. If possible, slightly less contrast than usual should be used.

Slice Thickness: 1.5 mm or 2 mm for menisci, 3 mm for patella alignment. For tumours 5 mm scans can be used.

Slice Incrementation: Contiguous slices.

Field of View: If a single knee, 16 cm. If both knees, 24–32 cm, depending on size of patient and proximity of the knees. Bone algorithm for patella alignment and bony tumours, otherwise a normal algorithm. High-resolution scan, especially for the menisci.

I.V. Contrast: Not usually required.

Window Settings: For menisci without an arthrogram: WW 200 HU, WL 70 HU. For bony lesions: WW 3200 HU, WL 200 HU. For soft tissue: WW 400 HU, WL 40 HU.

LARYNX

Patient Preparation

Nil by mouth for 2 h before.

Patient Position

Patient supine with arms by the sides. Scans performed on quiet breathing. The patient should not swallow during the scan, as this creates movement artefact. Scans can be taken through the vocal cords on phonation or suspended respiration to assess cord mobility.

Scan Parameters

Lateral scanogram (Fig. 19). Scan from angle of jaw to sternal notch, with a straight gantry.

Slice Thickness: 5 mm.

Slice Incrementation: 5 mm through larynx, 7 mm to sternal notch. If reformatted or 3-D images are to be obtained, keep incrementation at 5 mm.

Field of View: 16 cm. May have to increase to 18 cm, depending on patient. Remember not to rezoom if reformatted images are to be obtained. A low-dose body

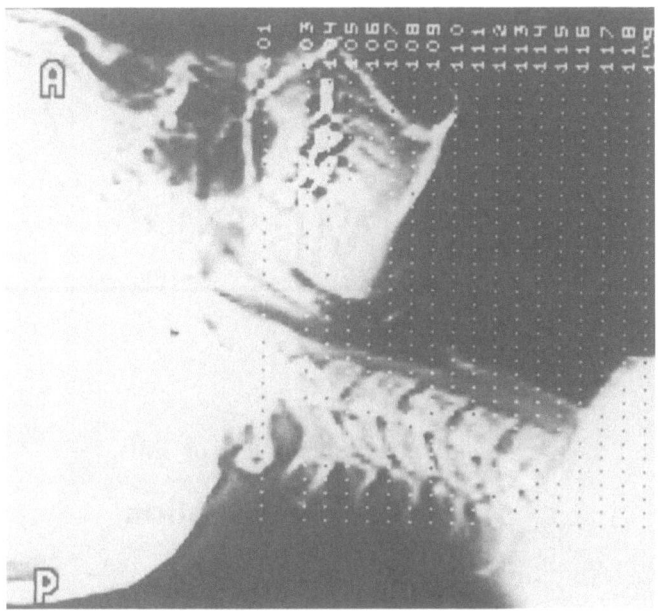

Fig. 19 Lateral scout. Scan from the angle of the jaw to the sternal notch.

scan is advisable. An infant headset (no calcium correction) may give better dosimetry.

I.V. Contrast: For laryngeal cancer, scans are taken during contrast infusion to help identification of nodes and vessels, unless specifically requested not to, e.g. for patients with severe respiratory compromise. 50–100 ml of non-ionic contrast is used. Inject 25–50 ml as a bolus to opacify the vessels, with the remainder injected during dynamic incremental scanning. If the scanner cannot perform enough scans before tube cooling becomes a problem, then use multiple smaller boluses of contrast. For laryngeal trauma i.v. contrast is not usually required, and 3-D imaging is recommended.

Window Settings: WW 400 HU, WL 40 HU.

LIMBS

For tumours of legs or arms.

Patient Preparation

None.

Patient Position

Try to place the relevant limb in the centre of the field. For legs it is often helpful to have both included, for anatomic comparison. For arms: If the affected arm cannot be moved, scan with the arm at the side and the normal arm above the patient's head (Fig. 20). Have the patient off-centred in the gantry so that the affected arm is as near the centre of the field as possible. Alternatively, if the arm can be raised, scans should be performed with it above the patient's head, with the normal arm by the side. This should only be done if the scan plane will *not* pass through the patient's head and orbits, and is thus usually only for tumours below the elbow. Bone algorithm if bony rather than soft tissue tumour.

Slice Thickness: 5 mm.

Slice Incrementation: 5 mm, unless a very extensive tumour, when 8–10 mm incrementation may be used.

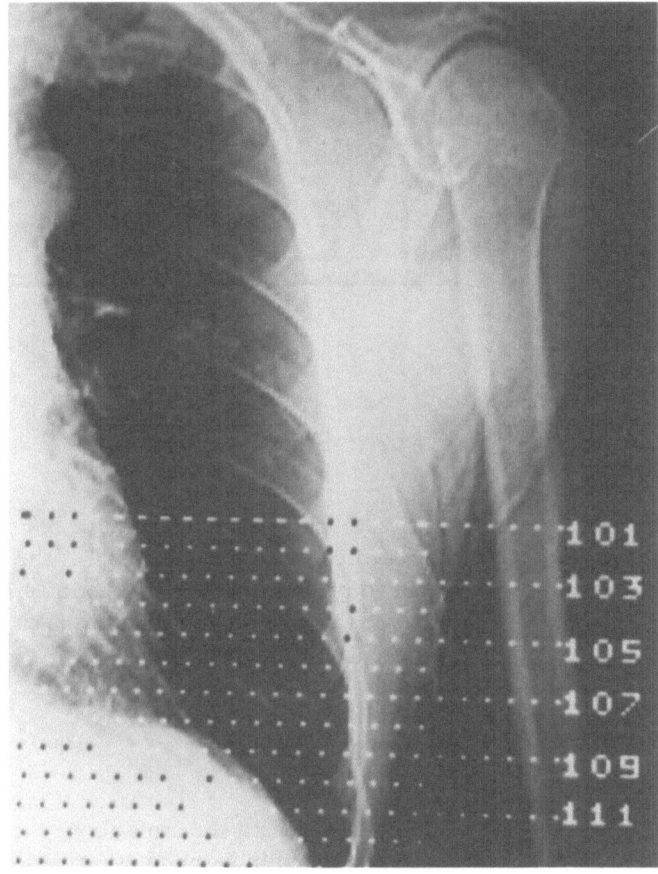

Fig. 20 AP scout. Scan through the affected area.

Field of View: 16, 24 or 32 cm, depending if one or both limbs are being scanned.

I.V. Contrast: Helpful in identifying vessels, especially in the leg. Give 50–100 ml while performing incremental dynamic scans. Start scanning at least 25 s after commencing the injection.

Window Settings: Soft tissue: WW 400 HU, WL 40 HU. Bone: WW 3200 HU, WL 200 HU.

LIVER

Patient Preparation

Nil by mouth for 4 h before. Oral contrast is given 30 min before, as for the abdomen. If the liver is the *only* organ to be scanned, the oral contrast can be omitted to decrease the artefact from the stomach, which can obscure small lesions in the liver.

Patient Position

Patient supine with the arms above the head. Scans should be taken in suspended expiration.

Scan Parameters

Frontal scanogram. Scan from top of diaphragm to bottom of liver or the aortic bifurcation, depending on the clinical problem (Fig. 21).

Slice Thickness: 10 mm.

Slice Incrementation: 10 mm if the liver is the organ of interest. 15 mm if part of a survey.

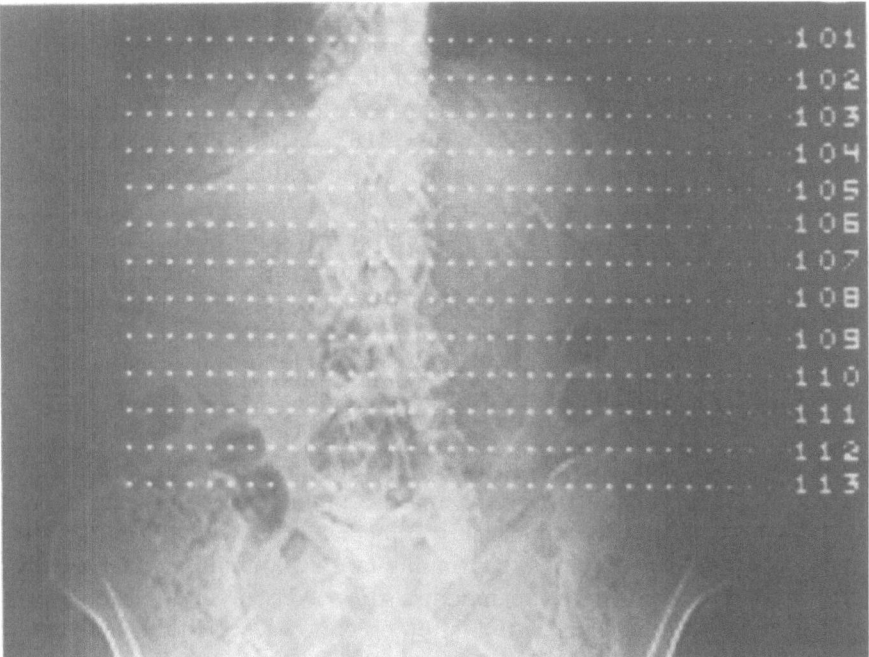

Fig. 21 AP scout. Scan from dome of diaphragm to L5.

Field of View: 32 cm or 40 cm.

I.V. Contrast: Usually unenhanced scans are performed initially, and contrast is given as below for
tumours, metastases and haemangiomas. Post-contrast
scans only can be performed for metastases, but some
vascular metastases may be missed. Unenhanced scans
should be performed initially, especially if fatty infiltra-
tion or haemochromatosis is to be identified.

There are many protocols for administering the i.v.
contrast, and below are some suggested methods. It
should be remembered that in the patient with known
malignant disease, with multiple solid lesions throughout the liver, metastases are the most likely diagnosis
and i.v. contrast may not be indicated at all.

Mass Lesions including metastases and hepatomas: 100 ml non-ionic contrast, 50 ml given as a bolus with the remainder given while incremental dynamic scanning is performed. Scanning should commence 20 s after the contrast injection is started, so that the portal vein is opacified. The whole liver should be scanned within 2–3 min to obtain the best contrast levels. If the scanner cannot scan the entire liver this quickly, then using larger volumes of more dilute contrast may be better. It is suggested that approximately 42 g of iodine needs to be administered to produce the best results. Delayed scans up to 4 h later may be helpful, but are usually logistically difficult.

Haemangiomas: Identify the abnormality on the unenhanced scan. Inject 50 ml contrast and scan the area of abnormality immediately, at 1 min, 2 min, 5 min and 10 min, continuing up to 30 min if necessary. Only 50% of haemangiomas show a classic CT appearance of a low attenuation lesion precontrast, which fills in from the periphery to the centre after i.v. contrast, becoming isodense on delayed scans.

Portal Vein Patency: As for mass lesions, or inject 50 ml of contrast as a bolus. Commence scan 20 s after injecting, and scan with 5 mm contiguous scans around portal vein.

Prior to Liver Resection: When it is important not only to know if metastases are present, but also how many and their position. A conventional CT scan has usually already been performed.

CT portography is considered the best method for detecting small, (less than 1 cm) lesions. An arterial catheter is positioned in the superior mesenteric artery under fluoroscopic control using the minimum amount of contrast. The patient is moved to the CT suite.

130 ml of dilute non-ionic contrast (200 mg/ml) are infused using a pump, at an infusion rate of 2 ml/s for 10 s, and the remainder at 1 ml/s. Contiguous 10 mm scans are taken from the dome of the diaphragm to the inferior margin of the liver, while the infusion is in progress. Scanning commences at the same time as the contrast infusion.

Hepatic artery and coeliac axis infusions do not give such reproducible results, due to variable hepatic artery anatomy.

Window Settings: WW 400 HU, WL 40 HU. It is also advantageous to view the images at a narrower window width of 200 HU, as this improves contrast resolution. If only hard copy is available the liver should be imaged on the two different windows.

NASOPHARYNX

Patient Preparation

Nil by mouth for 2 h before.

Patient Position

Supine with arms by side. Head in headrest with chin up. Scan on quiet respiration. Patient should not swallow during the scan as this causes motion artefact.

Scan Parameters

Lateral scanogram (Fig. 22). Scan from base of skull down to hyoid bone with a straight gantry. If the patient has a large amount of dental work causing artefact, a repeat scan with an angled gantry through the affected area may be helpful.

Slice Thickness: 5 mm.

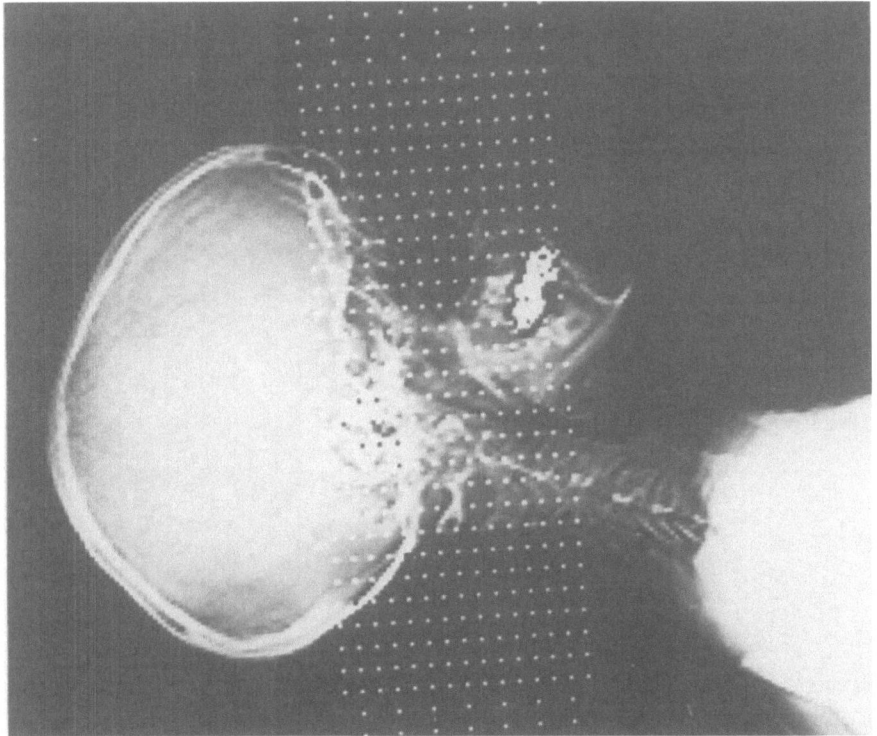

Fig. 22 Lateral scout. Scan from base of the skull to the hyoid.

Slice Incrementation: 5 mm through nasopharynx, 7 mm incrementation through remainder of neck if lymph nodes are to be staged.

Field of View: 16 cm. May need to be zoomed to 18 cm, depending on the size of the patient.

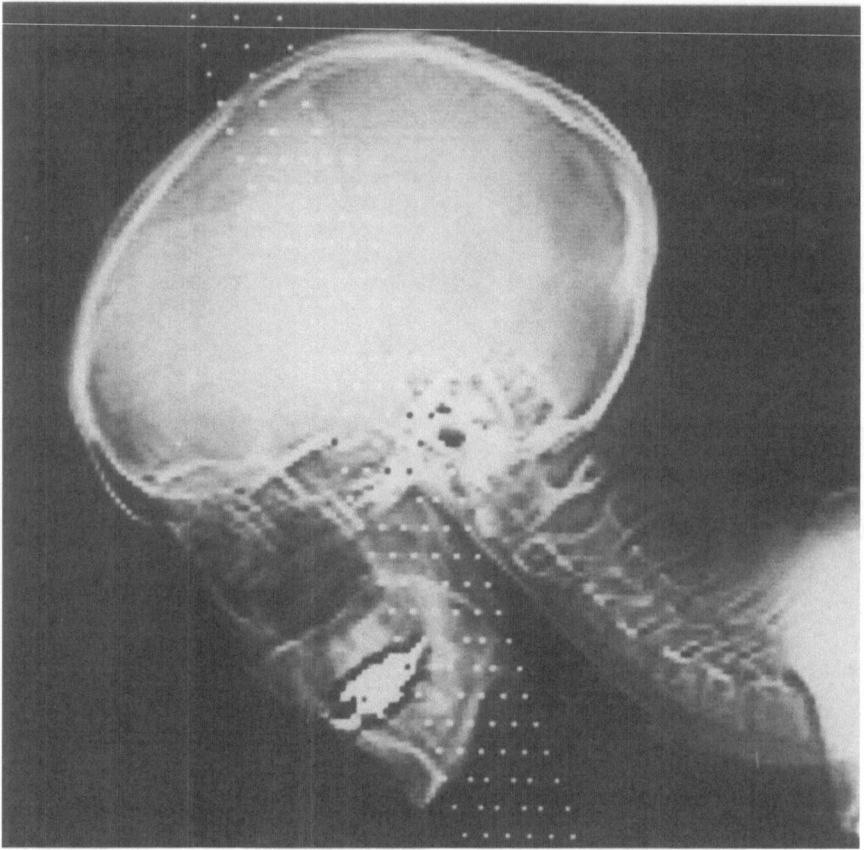

Fig. 23 Coronal scout. Scan through the nasopharynx.

I.V. Contrast: 50–100 ml of non-ionic contrast, 25–50 ml given a loading dose and the remainder injected during dynamic incremental scanning. If only the nasopharynx is to be scanned, 50 ml of contrast will probably be sufficient. Coronal scans may be helpful (Fig. 23). Patient prone or supine, depending on the headrest provided with the scanner. Lateral scanogram. First slice just anterior to the vertebral body, then scan anterior to this through the nasopharynx. Scan parameters as above.

Window Settings: WW 400 HU, WL 40 HU for soft tissues. To assess bony involvement of the base of the skull, WW 3200 HU, WL 200 HU. Narrowing the window down to 200–300 HU may improve contrast resolution.

Neck

Patient Preparation

Nil by mouth for 2 h before.

Patient Position

Patient supine with chin up and arms by the sides.
Scans performed on quiet breathing. Patient should not
swallow during the scan as this creates movement
artefact.

Scan Parameters

Lateral scanogram (Fig. 24). Scan from angle of jaw to
sternal notch, with a straight gantry.

Slice Thickness: 5 mm.

Slice Incrementation: 7 mm.

Field of View: 16 cm. May have to increase to 18 cm,
depending on patient. A low-dose body scan is advisable. An infant headset (no calcium correction) may give
better dosimetry.

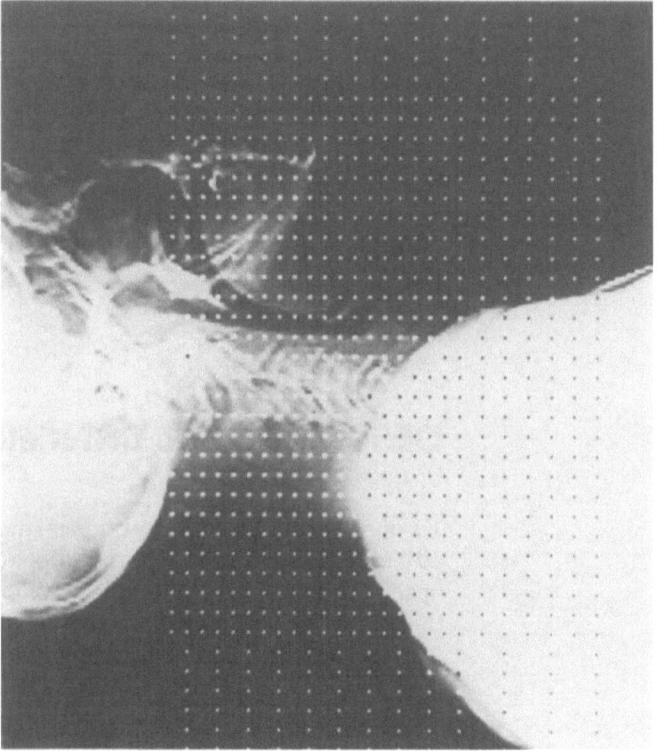

Fig. 24 Lateral scout. Scan from the angle of the jaw to the sternal notch.

I.V. Contrast: Scans are taken during contrast infusion to help identification of nodes and vessels. 50–100 ml of non-ionic contrast is used. Inject 25–50 ml as a bolus to opacify the vessels, with the remainder injected during dynamic incremental scanning. If the scanner cannot perform enough scans before tube cooling becomes a problem, then use multiple smaller boluses of contrast. For glomus tumours, scans can be limited to the area of interest.

Window Settings: WW 400 HU, WL 40 HU.

OESOPHAGUS

OESOPHAGEAL CANCER

To opacify the stomach and upper small bowel give
400 ml of oral contrast 30 min prior to the scan. To
opacify the oesophageal lumen, give oral contrast while
the patient is lying on the table immediately prior to
scanning. If the tumour is causing significant obstruction, two mouthfuls will be sufficient and will stay in the
lumen during the scan. If the oesophagus is not
obstructed the contrast will not remain, and the use of a
proprietary oesophageal contrast paste Esopho-Cat may
be advantageous. Scan from lung apices to bottom of
liver (Fig. 25).

Slice Thickness: 10 mm.

Slice Incrementation: 10 mm.

Field of View: 32 cm or 40 cm.

I.V. Contrast: 50–100 ml during incremental scanning in mediastinum and upper abdomen and liver if
required.

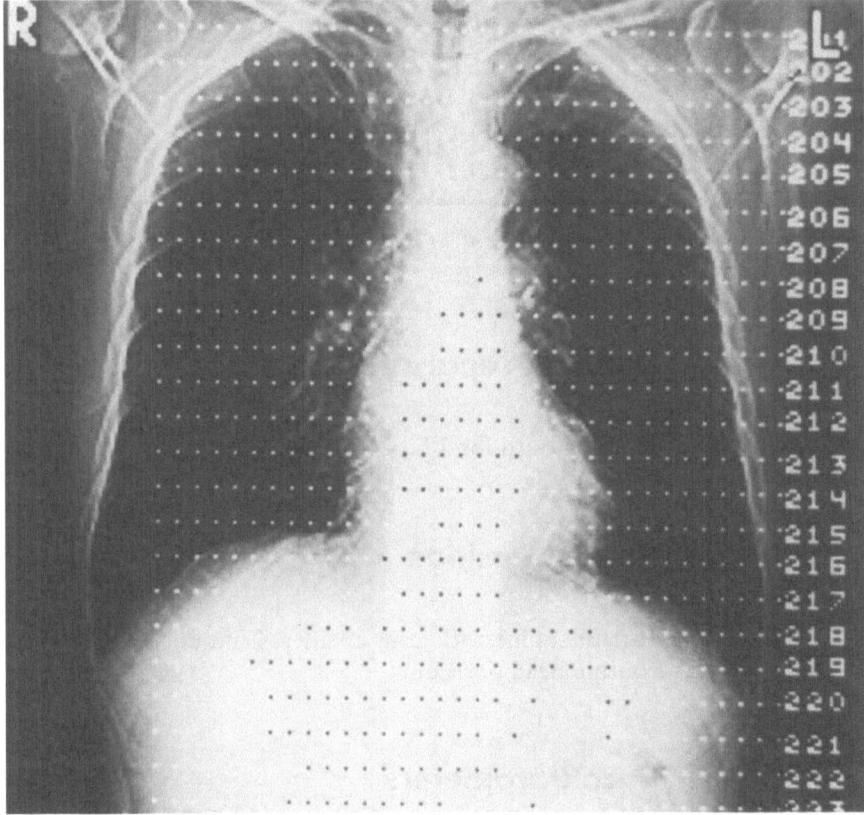

Fig. 25 AP scout. Scan from the apex or the lung to the bottom of the liver.

Window Settings: Lung parenchyma: WW 600–800 HU, WL –800 to –1000 HU. Mediastinum and abdomen: WW 400 HU, WL 40 HU.

ORBITS

Patient Preparation

Nil by mouth for 2 h before.

Patient Position

Patient supine with arms at sides. Chin raised from routine head position.

Scan Parameters

Lateral scanogram (Fig. 26). Scans should be taken parallel to the optic nerve. The plane of the scan is from the outer canthus of the eye to the anterior clinoid – always a positive angle. When scans are taken the patient should be asked to look upwards, to straighten the optic nerve and to keep the position of the eye constant. High-resolution scan.

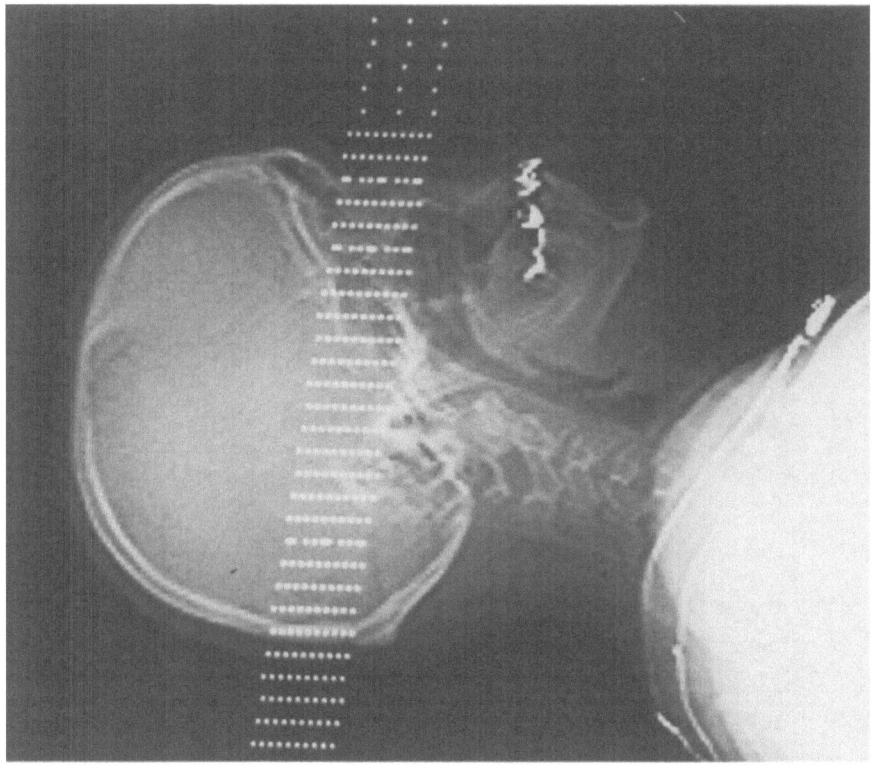

Fig. 26 Lateral scout. Scan parallel to the optic nerve (outer canthus to anterior clinoid).

Slice Thickness: 3 mm or 4 mm.

Slice Incrementation: 3 mm or 4 mm. Contiguous.

Field of View: 16 cm.

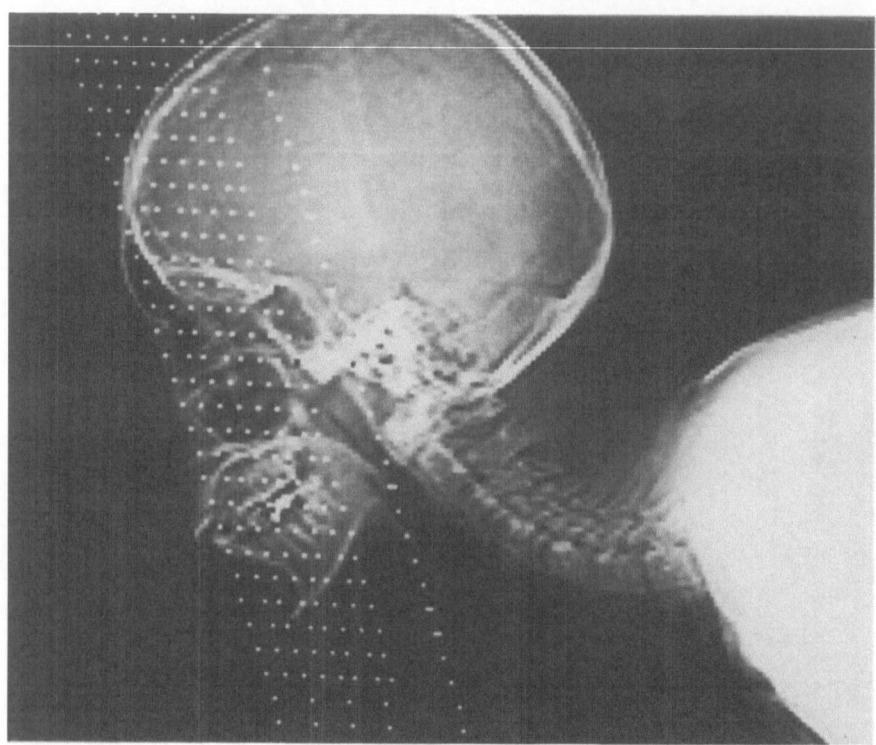

Fig. 27 Coronal scout. Scan posteriorly to level of cavernous sinus if necessary.

I.V. Contrast: CT delivers a large dose to the lens and therefore the number of scans should be limited. 50 ml of contrast can be given immediately prior to the scan. This will help in the identification of tumours or haemangiomas and may obviate the need for pre- and post-contrast scans, and thus decrease the dose to the lens.

Coronal Scans are often taken for orbital masses and may be continued posteriorly to the level of the cavernous sinus (Fig. 27). For patients with suspected thyroid eye disease, to determine the size of the muscles, coronal scans *only* may be obtained, which will avoid radiation to the lens. These patients do not require i.v. contrast.

Window Settings: WW 400 HU, WL 40 HU.

PANCREAS

Patient Preparation

Nil by mouth for 4 h before. Oral contrast as for abdomen. Rarely a scan without oral contrast may be performed if pancreatic calcification needs to be assessed, as the oral contrast may obscure faint calcification.

Patient Position

Supine with arms above head. Scan on suspended expiration. If the duodenal loop is not filled, turn the patient into the right lateral decubitus position which will fill it with contrast and improve visualisation of the head of the pancreas.

Scan Parameters

Frontal scanogram. The pancreas lies at about L1–L2 (Fig. 28). However, in most instances the abdomen will be scanned from the diaphragm down to the bifurcation.

Slice Thickness: 10 mm if a survey scan. For improved spatial resolution 5 mm scans should be obtained.

Scan Incrementation: 10 mm or 5 mm. Contiguous.

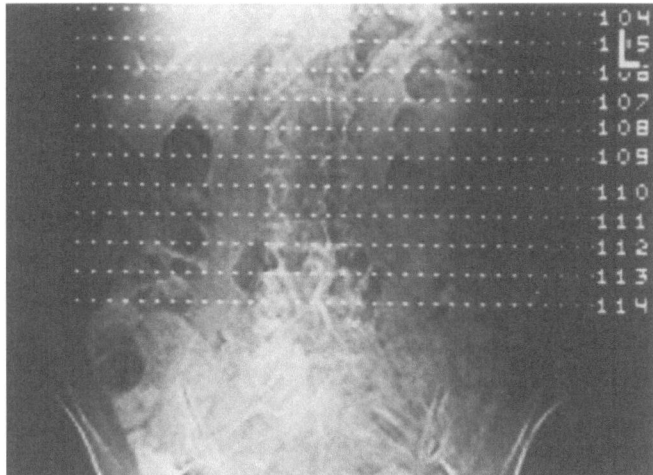

Fig. 28 AP Scout. Scan from T12 to L3.

Field of View: 32 cm or 40 cm. Use a 24 cm field of view if 5 mm slice used.

I.V. Contrast: 50–100 ml of non-ionic contrast. Inject 25–50 ml as a bolus and perform dynamic incremental scans through the pancreas while the remainder of the contrast is injected. Commence scanning 20–25 s after beginning the contrast.

Window Settings: WW 400 HU, WL 40 HU.

Pancreatitis: Scan 10 mm on 15 mm through the liver, 10 mm on 10 mm through the pancreas, and continue as far as necessary. Fluid collections may extend into the pelvis or into the chest. Pancreatic viability can be assessed by performing dynamic incremental scans through the pancreas after i.v. contrast, given as above.

Pancreatic Cancer: The normal pancreas enhances and pancreatic tumours normally enhance less well, and are better defined after contrast. Dynamic incremental scans should be performed, which should include the liver if looking for metastases, and down to the bifurcation for para-aortic nodes.

PARATHYROIDS

Patient Preparation

Nil by mouth for 2 h before.

Patient Position

Supine with arms by sides. Scans taken on quiet breathing. Patient should not swallow during the scans.

Scan Parameters

Frontal scanogram of neck and upper chest (Fig. 29). Scan from the cricoid down to the sternal notch without contrast, and from the cricoid to the bottom of the aortic arch post-contrast. Scans with a higher mA may be needed to obtain good views through the shoulders.

Slice Thickness: 5 mm.

Slice Incrementation: 5 mm.

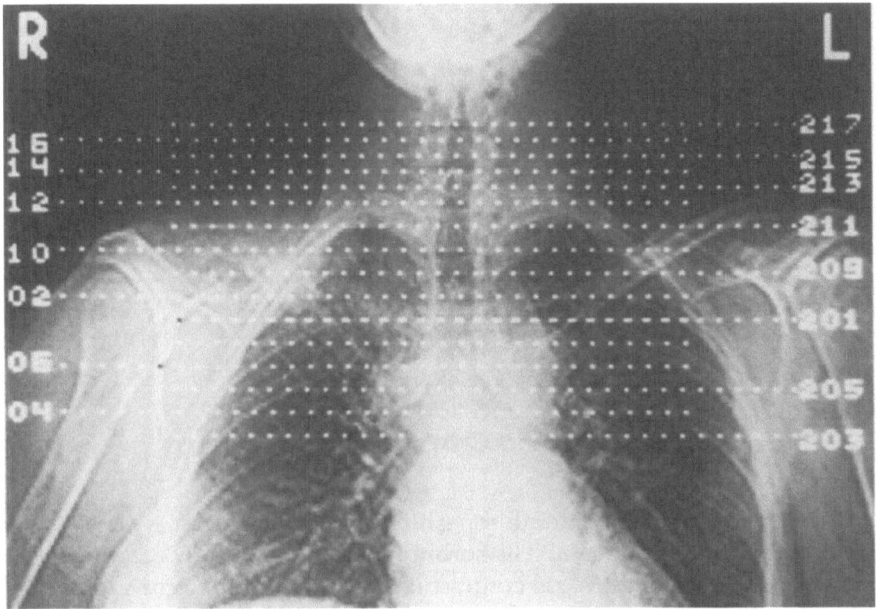

Fig. 29 AP scout. Scan from cricoid to aortic arch.

Field of View: 16 cm.

I.V. Contrast: 50–100 ml non-ionic contrast, 25–50 ml as a bolus and the remainder during the scans. Dynamic incremental scans from the cricoid down to the bottom of arch of the aorta, to look for ectopic parathyroid tissue.

Window Settings: WW 400 HU, WL 40 HU. It may be helpful to view on WW of 200 HU.

PELVIS

Patient Preparation

Nil by mouth for 4 h before. Oral contrast – see abdomen. The sorbitol mixture is strongly recommended. Rectal contrast if indicated. Tampon for vagina may be helpful.

Patient Position

Supine with arms above head if the abdomen and pelvis are both to be scanned, or arms across chest if only the pelvis is to be scanned. Quiet or suspended respiration.

Scan Parameters

Frontal scanogram (Fig. 30) to include abdomen and pelvis if necessary. Scan from pubic symphysis to top of iliac crest.

Slice Thickness: 10 mm if survey, 5 mm for improved spatial resolution.

Slice Incrementation: 5 or 10 mm. Contiguous.

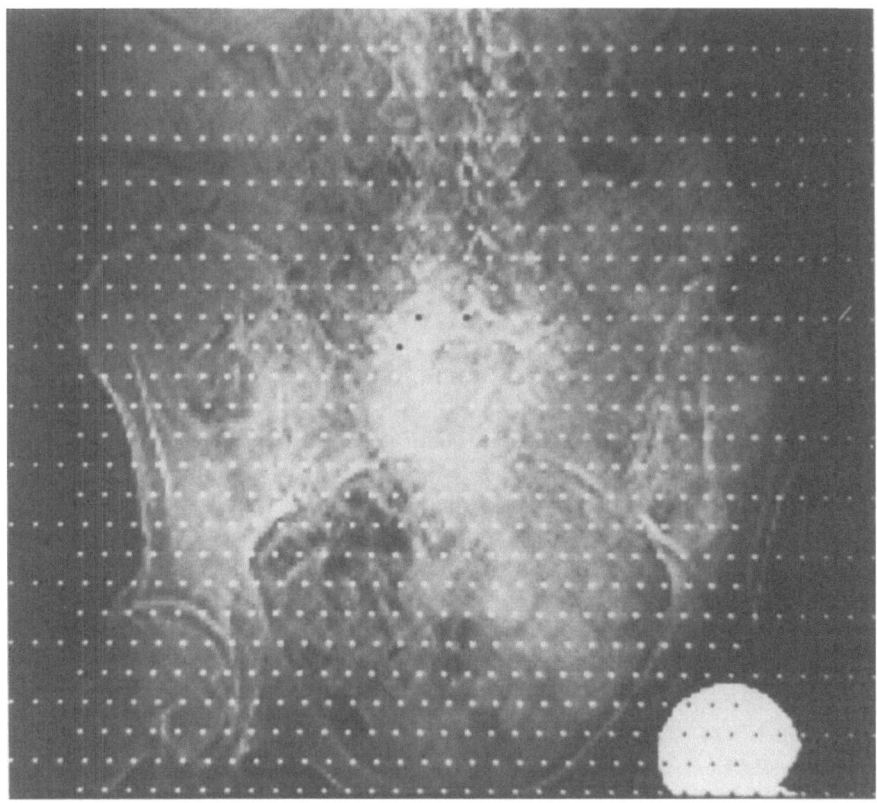

Fig. 30 AP scout. Scan from pubic symphysis to iliac crest.

Field of View: 32 cm or 40 cm.

I.V. Contrast: To identify the iliac vessels and differentiate them from nodes, use 50–100 ml of non-ionic contrast, 25–50 ml as a bolus and the remainder given during dynamic incremental scanning through the pelvis, starting at the pubic symphysis and scanning craniad. Commence scanning at least 25 s after the beginning of the injection, to allow the contrast time to reach the iliac vessels.

RECTAL CANCER

Oral Contrast: As above.

Slice Thickness: 10 mm.

Slice Incrementation: 10 mm through the pelvis. 15 mm to the liver and 10 mm through the liver.

Field of View: 32 or 40 cm.

I.V. Contrast: As above.

Window Settings: WW 400 HU, WL 40 HU.

CANCER OF CERVIX AND OVARY

As for rectal cancer.

PITUITARY

Patient Preparation

Nil by mouth for 2 h before.

Patient Position

Scans can be performed either in the transaxial or the coronal plane. Transaxial scans can be reformatted into coronal or sagittal planes. Transaxial scans require multiple scans to be taken through the lens, therefore to reduce the dose to the lens coronal scans should be obtained and reformatted in the transaxial or sagittal planes. *Coronal scans:* patient prone or supine depending on the headrest provided. The neck should be fully extended with the chin forward to keep any dental amalgam out of the sections. *Transaxial scans:* patient supine with the chin up.

Scan Parameters

Lateral scanogram. For coronal scans, scan from the posterior to anterior clinoids with the plane of the scan perpendicular to the floor of the fossa (Fig. 31). For transaxial scans, scan with a straight gantry from below the floor of the sella to above the clinoids (Fig. 32).

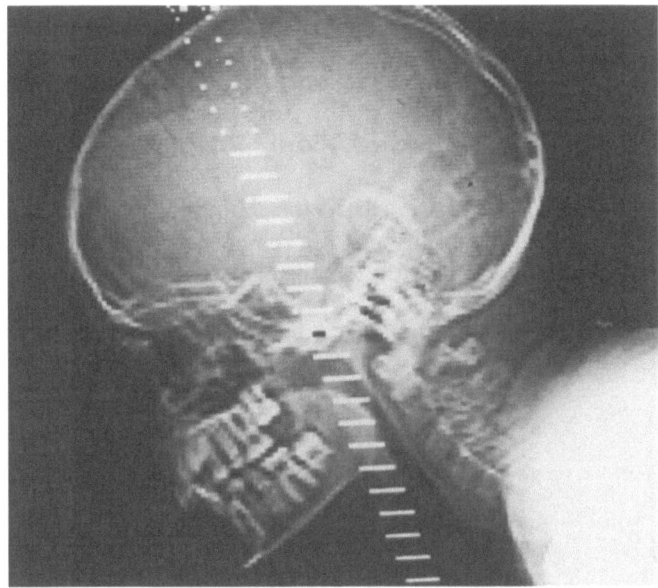

Fig. 31 Coronal scout. Scan from posterior to anterior clinoids.

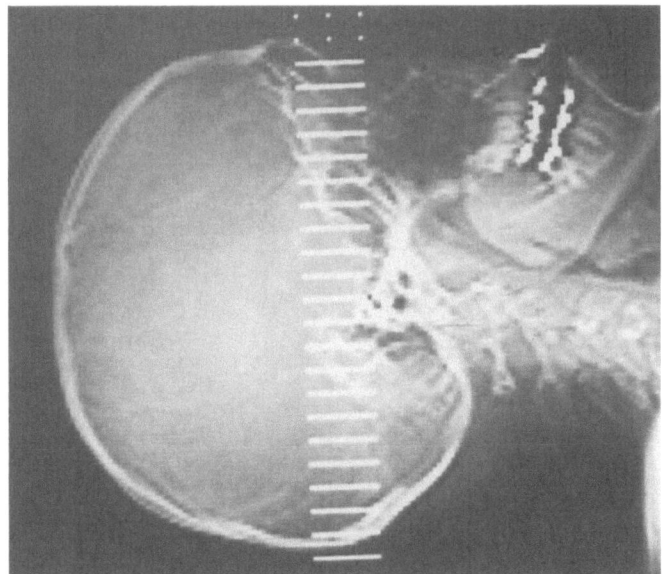

Fig. 32 Lateral scout. Scan from sphenoid sinus to above clinoids.

Slice Thickness: 2 mm. High precision.

Slice Incrementation: 2 mm. Contiguous.

Field of View: 16 cm. May zoom to 12 cm.

I.V. Contrast: 100 ml non-ionic contrast, 50 ml as a bolus and the remainder while dynamic incremental scanning is performed.

Window Settings: WW 200–250 HU, WL 50 HU.

Transaxial Scans: For patients unable to maintain coronal position, or at the request of the radiologist. Raise the chin so there is less artefact from petrous bone. Start scans below the floor of the fossa. Scan parameters as above.

SACROILIAC JOINTS

Patient Preparation

None. No oral contrast.

Patient Position

Supine with the arms across the chest.

Scan Parameters

Frontal scanogram of the pelvis (Fig. 33). Scan through the sacroiliac joints. Both joints to be visualised. Bone algorithm. Alternatively use a lateral scanogram and angle the gantry parallel to the sacroiliac joints (Fig. 34).

Slice Thickness: 5 mm.

Slice Incrementation: 5 mm. Contiguous.

Field of View: 24 cm.

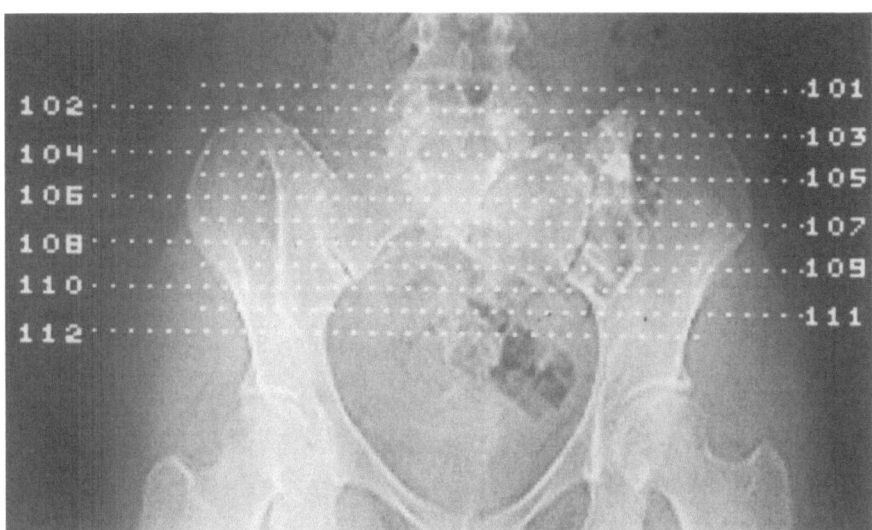

Fig. 33 AP scout. Scan from top to bottom of joints.

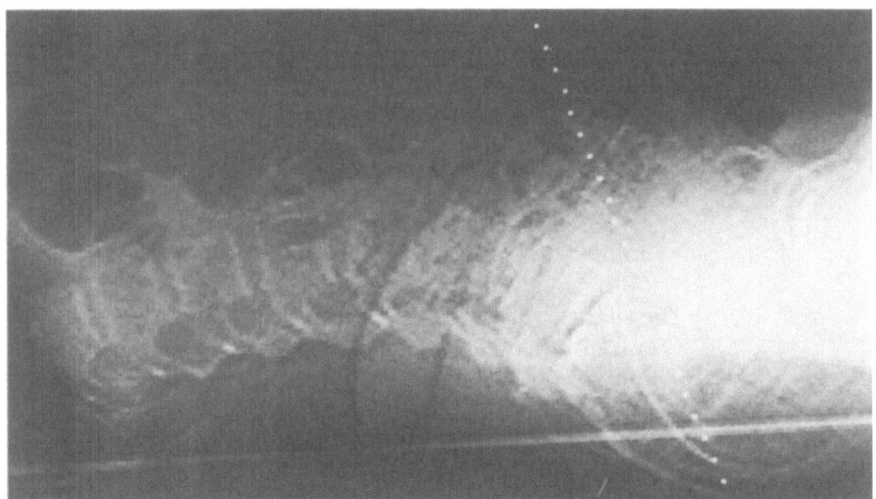

Fig. 34 Lateral scout. Angle gantry parallel to sacrum and scan posteriorly.

I.V. Contrast: Not required.

Window Settings: Bone: WW 3200 HU, WL 200 HU. Soft tissue: WW 400 HU, WL 40 HU.

SHOULDERS

Patient Preparation

None if the scan is to look for intra-articular loose bodies. If the scan is to assess the labrum it should be performed after a double contrast shoulder arthrogram, using slightly less contrast than usual. Some authors suggest using as little as 1 ml of contrast with 10–12 ml of air.

Patient Position

Supine, with the arms by the sides in the neutral position or in minimal internal rotation. The patient should be slightly off-centre, so that the shoulder is as near the centre of the field as possible. Scan on suspended respiration. Scanning the patient prone may provide better visualisation of the labrum when the scan is performed in conjunction with a double-contrast arthrogram.

Scan Parameters

Frontal chest scanogram (Fig. 35). Scan from the mid-acromioclavicular joint to the inferior surface of the glenoid.

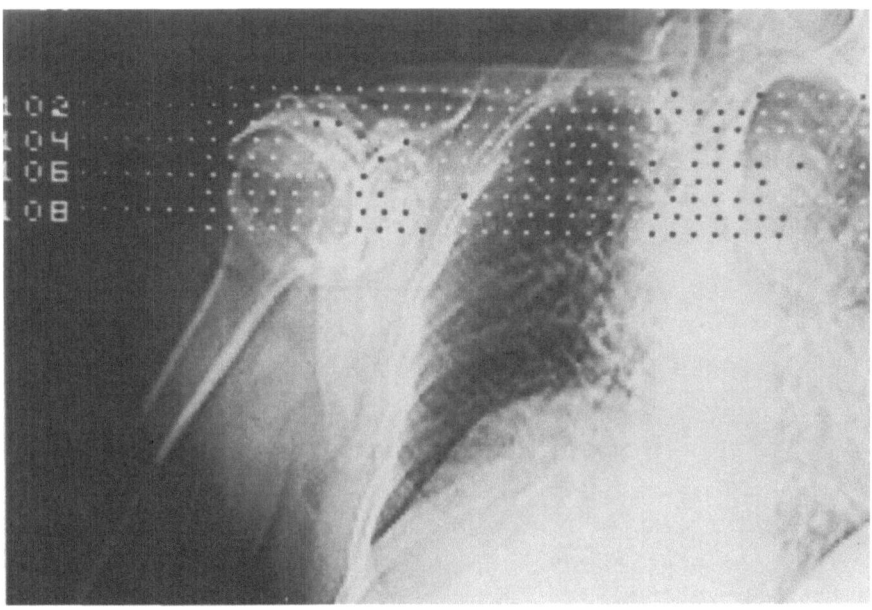

Fig. 35 AP scout. Scan from mid-acromioclavicular joint to bottom of glenoid.

Scan Thickness: 3 mm or 5 mm. Precision scan.

Slice Incrementation: Contiguous.

Field of View: 16 cm.

I.V. Contrast: Not required; intra-articular contrast if necessary – see above.

Window Settings: WW 2000 HU, WL 250 HU.

Spine

Patient Preparation

None.

Patient Position

Supine with the arms across the chest.

Scan Parameters

If no plain films, do anteroposterior and lateral scanograms, to check the number of vertebrae.

Slice Thickness: 3 mm. High-precision scan. Filter 5.

Slice Incrementation: 3 mm. Contiguous.

Field of View: 16 cm. Zoom to 12 cm.

I.V. Contrast: Not usually required.

Window Settings: Soft tissue: WW 600 HU, WL 100 HU. Bone: WW 3200 HU, WL 200 HU.

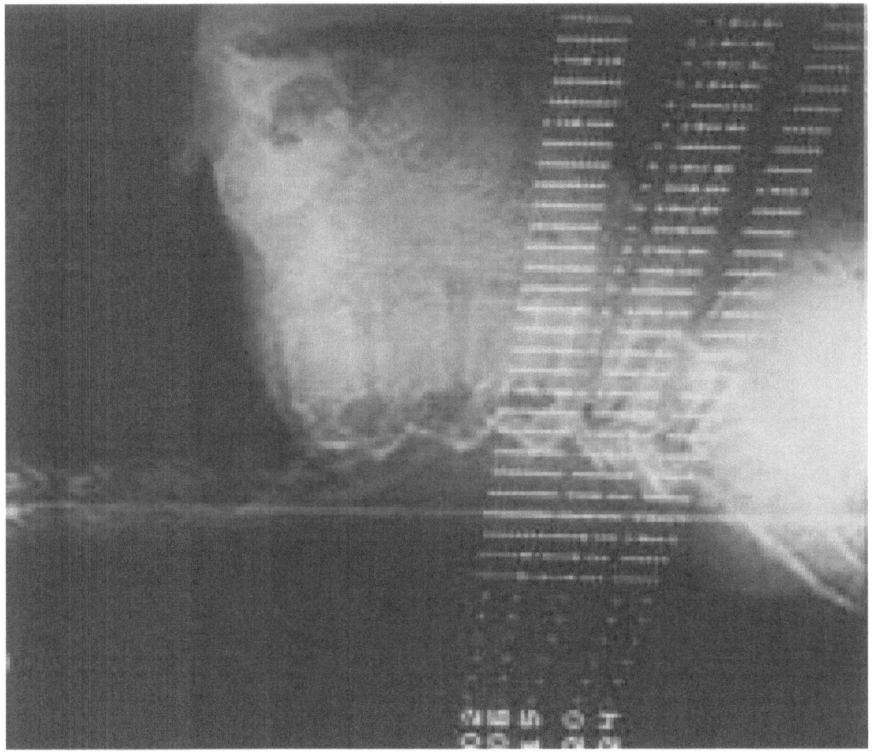

Fig. 36 Lateral scout. Angle gantry and scan from inferior to superior pedicle.

LUMBAR SPINE

Lumbar Disc: Angle gantry parallel to the end plate (Fig. 36). Contiguous slices from pedicle to pedicle through the lower three disc spaces.

Spines for Reformatting: Use the above parameters but with a straight gantry. Scan from pedicles of L3 or L4 to S1. Do not zoom image. Do not move image around screen. Scan parameters as above.

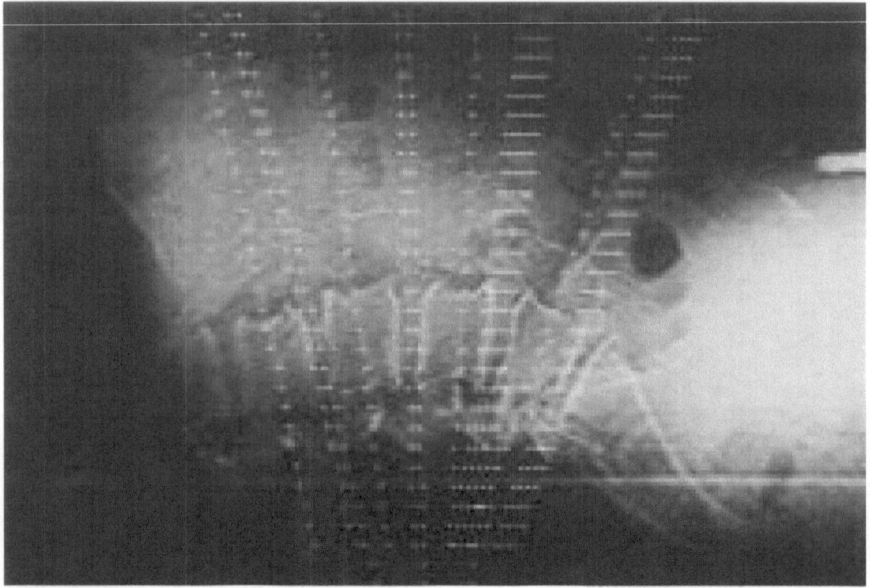

Fig. 37 Lateral scout. Angle gantry and scan through mid-body and disc space of each vertebra.

Spinal Canal Stenosis: Angle gantry parallel to the end plate. 1 scan through pedicle, 2 through disc. Scan from L2–S1 (Fig. 37). Scan parameters as above. Remember to put vertebral levels on scan.

Spinal Trauma: It is better to use a straight gantry and contiguous slices as above, so that reformatting can be undertaken.

Post-myelogram: Either a straight or angled gantry and the above scan parameters. If a large area needs to be scanned, then a 5 mm slice thickness may be preferable, depending on the clinical problem. The images are viewed on a wider window than usual. Postoperative spines may need i.v. contrast – give 100 ml, 50 ml as a bolus and the remaining 50 ml while performing dynamic incremental scans. Fibrosis enhances, and prolapsed disc material does not.

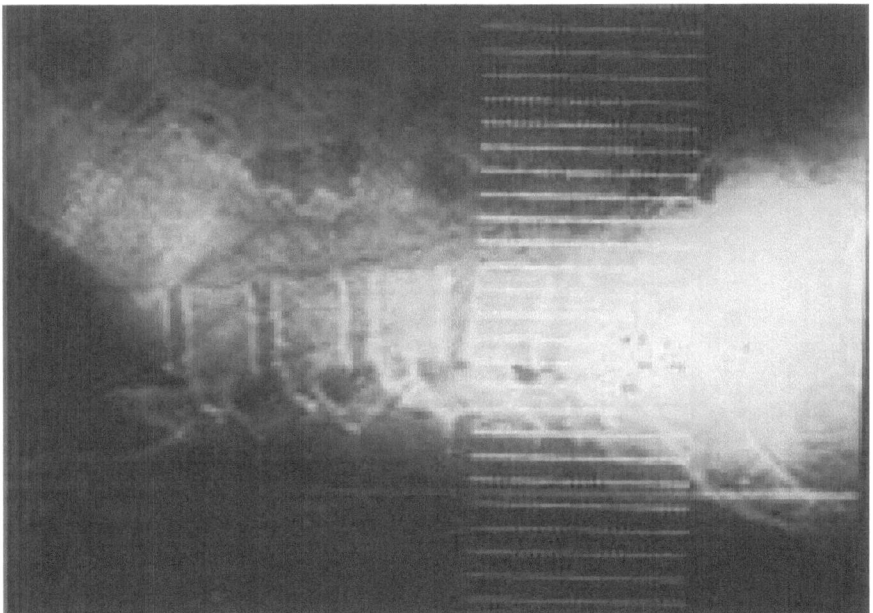

Fig. 38 Straight gantry. Can use AP or lateral scout.

Spondylolisthesis: If the gantry angulation is not sufficient to scan through the L5/S1 disc parallel to the end plates, then use contiguous scans with a straight gantry which can then be reformatted (Fig. 38). These scans can be reformatted in any plane.

THORACIC AND CERVICAL SPINE

Trauma: As above.

Disc Disease: Cervical discs may be seen without intrathecal contrast, but intrathecal contrast is advisable if the level of the disc is unknown, to avoid scanning the entire cervical spine with thin-section high-dose scans.

Spinal Tumours: Intrathecal contrast *must* be administered. For diagnosis of a syrinx a scan at 24 h may be helpful.

WINDOWS

Abdomen: WW 300 or 400, WL 30 or 40.

Brain: WW 150, WL 36 (posterior fossa); WW 75, WL 36 (Remainder of head). WW 3200, WL 200 (petrous bones).

Chest: WW 300 or 400, WL 35 or 40 (mediastinum); WW 600, WL –750 (lungs).

Facial Bones: WW 600, WL 100.

IAMs: WW 3200, WL 200 (coronals), WL 100 (transaxials).

Neck: WW 400, WL 40.

Pituitary: WW 200, WL 50.

Orbits: WW 400, WL 50.

Pelvis: WW 300 or 400, WL 30 or 40.

Sinuses: WW 1600 or 3200, WL 200.

Spine: WW 600, WL 100.

Spine Post-myelogram (soft tissue): 3 h: WW 800, WL 150. 24 h: WW 300 (cervical spine), 400 (thoracic spine), WL 40.

Suggested Reading

Brooke JR (1989) CT and Somography of the acute abdomen. Raven Press

Grainger R, Allison D (1992) Diagnostic radiology (2nd edn). Churchill Livingstone, London

Lee J, Sagel S, Stanley R (1991) Computed body tomography with MRI correlation (2nd edn), Raven, New York

Moss A, Gamsu G, Genant H (1991) Computed tomography of the body (2nd edn). Saunders, Philadelphia

Williams A, Haughton V (1985) Cranial computed tomography. A comprehensive text. CV Mosby